T0231728

Ethics and Values
in Long Term Health Care

Ethics and Values in Long Term Health Care

Patricia J. Villani, PhD, MPA
Editor

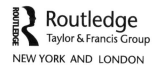

Routledge
Taylor & Francis Group
NEW YORK AND LONDON

First published 1994 by The Haworth Press,Inc.,
The Haworth Press, Inc., 10 Alice Street, Binghamton, NY 13904-1580 USA

This edition Published 2016 by Routledge
711 Third Avenue, New York, NY 10017, USA
2 Park Square, Milton Park, Abingdon, Oxon OX14 4RN

Routledge is an imprint of the Taylor & Francis Group, an informa business

Ethics and Values in Long Term Health Care has also been published as *Activities, Adaptation & Aging*, Volume 18, Numbers 3/4 1994.

Library of Congress Cataloging-in-Publication Data

Ethics and values in long term health care / Patricia J. Villani, editor.
    p.   cm.
    "Has also been published as: Activities, adaptation & aging, volume 18, numbers 3/4, 1994"–T.p. verso.
    Includes bibliographical references.
    ISBN 1-56024-698-7 (alk. paper)
    1. Aged–Long-term care–Moral and ethical aspects. I. Villani, Patricia J.
    [DNLM: 1. Ethics, Medical. 2. Long-Term Care. 3. Caregivers. 4. Music Therapy. 5. Health Care Reform. W 50 E8413 1994]
RC954.3.E87 1994
174'.2–dc20
DNLM/DLC
for Library of Congress
    94-35455
    CIP

ISBN 13: 978-1-56024-698-5 (hbk)

Ethics and Values
in Long Term Health Care

CONTENTS

CAREGIVING

END OF LIFE CHOICES

HEALTH CARE REFORM

ABOUT THE EDITOR

Patricia J. Villani, PhD, MPA, is President of Gerontology for Education and Research Opportunities, Inc. (GERO, Inc.), a consulting firm that assists public and private organizations in planning, implementing, and expanding quality eldercare programs. Her 22 years of experience as a program planner and program director in the U.S. Public Health Service, combined with her years as a private consultant, have given Dr. Villani a broad-based knowledge of health care systems. She has had the opportunity to appraise and analyze ethical dilemmas in many types of health care settings. Dr. Villani is also the Administrator of the Washington Area Geriatric Education Center Consortium in Washington, DC.

Foreword

Ethical dilemmas for health practitioners working with older persons have been researched and discussed for many years. Conflicts in ethics and values emerge from factors that are both personal and professional. Opposing values tend to create myriad ethical dilemmas for the practitioner. These ethical quandaries often have a direct impact on services to the aging consumer.

Documented in this volume are a variety of ethics and values concerns spanning approaches within the emerging health care reform environment to dilemmas regarding end of life choices. The views presented by no means encompass all aspects of the ethical challenges facing health care practitioners today. Rather this effort informs practitioners of some of the more basic dilemmas and issues they continue to face in a host of health care services environments. Where possible, practical and philosophical, as well as ethical, perspectives have been explored. It is hoped that the information presented will be used as a catalyst for innovative thinking and a guide for positive action for all readers.

Thomas M. Ennis

[Haworth co-indexing entry note]: "Foreword," Ennis, Thomas M. Co-published simultaneously in *Activities, Adaptation & Aging* (The Haworth Press, Inc.) Vol. 18, No. 3/4, 1994, p. xiii; and: *Ethics and Values in Long Term Health Care* (ed: Patricia J. Villani) The Haworth Press, Inc., 1994, p. xiii. Multiple copies of this article/chapter may be purchased from The Haworth Document Delivery Center [1-800-3-HAWORTH; 9:00 a.m. - 5:00 p.m. (EST)].

Introduction

Since the 1940s, ethical issues for practitioners in eldercare have become a growing concern as we continue to strive toward maintaining the welfare of those in our care. Various monitoring mechanisms and codes of conduct and ethics designed for specific disciplines have evolved to ensure that guidelines are in place to resolve dilemmas. However, we know that ethical choices are made based on an individual's awareness and interpretation of these mechanisms and codes. We also are aware that in many instances, societal guides do not go far enough and are not clear enough to help us resolve these ethical conflicts.

Although defining right and wrong is often the product of an individual's upbringing or stems from a professional code of ethics, few health practitioners have received formal training in value assessment or in appropriate analysis of ethical enigmas. As eldercare practitioners, we must work together to find the appropriate balance between human rights and values and the objectives of our professions. It is crucial that we do not neglect these issues–the result may be that ethics for our professions will be "enforced" through regulation, putting unrealistic limitations on us with no allowances for creativity or moral discretion.

It is important that we continue to listen, learn, and be diligent in our efforts to tackle new challenges in ethical conduct. Readers are encouraged to relate the lessons contained in this journal to practical decision-making in their respective health profession. Through information and discussion, we can develop new modes of ethical

[Haworth co-indexing entry note]: "Introduction," Villani, Patricia J. Co-published simultaneously in *Activities, Adaptation & Aging* (The Haworth Press, Inc.) Vol. 18, No. 3/4, 1994, pp. 1-2; and: *Ethics and Values in Long Term Health Care* (ed: Patricia J. Villani) The Haworth Press, Inc., 1994, pp. 1-2. Multiple copies of this article/chapter may be purchased from The Haworth Document Delivery Center [1-800-3-HAWORTH; 9:00 a.m. - 5:00 p.m. (EST)].

1

thinking that will enhance practice as we improve the quality of the lives of the elderly. We will then be ready to confront some of the major ethics and values challenges during the 1990s and beyond.

Patricia J. Villani

PRACTITIONER KNOWLEDGE

A Beginner's Guide to Ethical Awareness in Long-Term Care Services

Priscilla Kimboko
Eva Jewell

SUMMARY. This article provides a basic overview of key ethical concepts relevant to long-term care. It recommends steps to follow in establishing an ethics committee in long-term care settings. The purpose of such a committee is to assist professionals and decision makers in evaluating the choices and decisions they face in their own long-term care or aging service setting on a daily basis. Case studies are included as an appendix to the article to illustrate ethical concepts and dimensions and to provide a new group with starting points for ethical discussions.

THE CONTEXT FOR ETHICAL DILEMMAS OF LONG-TERM CARE

Health and human service professionals have shown a growing interest and attention to the ethical aspects of long-term care in recent years. The trend to deal with "ethics" in care began with

---

Priscilla Kimboko, PhD, is Assistant Dean, University of Northern Colorado Graduate School, Greeley, CO, and continues to teach courses in gerontology at the school.

Eva Jewell, MA, is Long Term Care Administrator, Weld Area Agency on Aging, Greeley, CO. Ms. Jewell also teaches graduate courses in gerontology and participates in research activities at the University of Northern Colorado.

[Haworth co-indexing entry note]: "A Beginner's Guide to Ethical Awareness in Long-Term Care Services," Kimboko, Priscilla, and Eva Jewell. Co-published simultaneously in *Activities, Adaptation & Aging* (The Haworth Press, Inc.) Vol. 18, No. 3/4, 1994, pp. 5-26; and: *Ethics and Values in Long Term Health Care* (ed: Patricia J. Villani) The Haworth Press, Inc., 1994, pp. 5-26. Multiple copies of this article/chapter may be purchased from The Haworth Document Delivery Center [1-800-3-HAWORTH; 9:00 a.m. - 5:00 p.m. (EST)].

5

medical professionals in acute care settings who were seeking to address the many dilemmas they face in providing appropriate care, given the interface of sophisticated life-prolonging technologies and the increasing age and activism of patients. Such ethical conflicts and dilemmas in the acute care setting are routinely addressed through the auspices of the biomedical ethics committee, now present in most hospital settings.

More recently professionals in other domains of care to the elderly and disabled, including nursing home, home care, and managed care providers and settings, find themselves confronting many similar conflicts regarding the proper nature and type of care and the role of the clients, family members and professionals in deciding on appropriate care. Conflicts often revolve around who has the right to choose (or refuse) different services and related options, and to decide on behalf of individuals about questions of when and how an individual will live or die. While there have been many recent legal or regulatory decisions that impact on professionals providing care in nursing homes, private homes, and community-care settings, the legal responses are not always equivalent to the ethical response. Ethical issues are often more complex questions about what is the right or wrong thing to do, even within the legal options.

In their day to day encounters with clients, families, and professional colleagues, a human service or health professional cannot avoid questions about right and wrong (Downie and Calman, 1987). How people define right and wrong is often a function of their own personal values or their own profession's code of ethics. Few professionals engaged in long-term care service delivery have received formal training in ethics, which allows them to assess and evaluate decisions or actions of others in a larger framework of ethical decisions. By the very nature of long-term care, however, no one profession is prepared to meet all the service needs of the clients. Multiple professions must work together. Yet, the professional codes which guide the practice of different professionals are often contradictory and incomplete, particularly when it comes to issues of conflicts among professionals and clients regarding health and social service needs and options.

Confronted with such ongoing daily dilemmas, professionals in long-term care services often experience "burn-out," skepticism, despair, and anger. These are normal responses to the stress of dealing with life and death issues, with confronting conflicts in values and beliefs, and with realizing that resource limitations and regulations prevent doing all that one's professional judgment demands.

It is important to the well-being of professionals and clients in the long-term care system, that such issues get addressed collectively rather than individually. More and more community service providers and nursing homes are adopting the bioethics committee model of hospitals to more effectively address these moral and ethical issues in long-term care.

The purpose of this paper is to provide some guidance to those who are interested in beginning such a committee in their facility or community. In this paper we review some of the basic moral concepts and rules to establish the basis for the common language required for persons working together in the broad medical-social context of long-term care. We suggest some ways that professionals can effectively articulate their thoughts and feelings about moral issues. We discuss the nature, purpose, development and operating procedures of an ethics committee, with some precautionary observations provided about possible pitfalls in this process. And, finally, we present several case studies in which we begin to use this common ethical language, to illustrate the types of issues an ethics "group" would face.

STRATEGIES FOR RESOLVING MORAL DILEMMAS IN LONG-TERM CARE

Resolving the moral dilemmas which arise in long-term care services requires professionals to have a forum for an open and frank discussion of the contradictions, conflicts, and differences in values that they confront in their interdependent daily caregiving decisions. In order to resolve dilemmas, it is important that caregivers from different professions have "a systematic, principled manner of clarifying the issues (Denver Community Bioethics Committee, 1993) and that they have a dialogue about ethical choices and actions. Abramson (1985) suggested the following guidelines for beginning such a dialogue:

1. All those working together must learn a common "moral" or "ethical" language dealing with the basic moral concepts and rules.
2. Members of the groups must "learn to articulate their thoughts and feelings about these important moral issues in ways that reduce the ambiguity . . . " (p. 37).
3. Group members should, individually and as a group, spend time clarifying and prioritizing values and moral principles.
4. The group should have regular procedures for analyzing complex ethical dilemmas when they arise.

In a similar vein, the American Association for Retired Persons (AARP, 1990) suggests that institutions and agencies in the long-term care system can benefit from a well-conceived ethics committee. In a brochure on this topic, they suggest that an important first step is to form an ad hoc group to list the problematic issues and cases that raise moral or ethical concerns, to develop a mission statement regarding the need for and purpose of the ethics committee, and then to develop the plan, to include membership, resource needs and specific operational guidelines.

DEVELOPING A COMMON LANGUAGE OF ETHICAL CONCEPTS

For the novice who has no prior experience in ethical discussions, and, particularly for professionals from diverse backgrounds whose professional codes of ethics differ in their assumptions, role definitions, and guiding principles, it is important and helpful to seek to establish a shared understanding of the principles and concepts that guide ethical practice. These concepts are briefly defined below, and are presented more from the perspective of the helping professional than from that of a philosopher. The goal is not to become philosophically "correct" and "erudite," but to use the concepts developed in ethics to enlighten our ability to identify and frame the dilemmas we face in the helping professions. As noted by Downie and Calman (1987), "development of moral consciousness requires more than reading a book . . . it requires active participation" (p. 4).

For purposes of this paper, ethics comprises a set of principles that should guide the actions of an individual, in deciding about issues of right and wrong actions, which arise in every-day encounters with "clients" and other care-providers. Ethics is the application of moral principles to daily practice decisions, to choice of action. Moral principles help people to live together harmoniously and cooperatively in society and help us distinguish between right and wrong actions.

There are four key moral principles that most ethicists and, in particular, most biomedical ethics committees, apply to the provision of medical and social care. These four principles are: (1) respect for autonomy, (2) beneficence/compassion, (3) nonmaleficence, and (4) justice. Derived from these four principles are several rules of ethical care provisions which should guide the professional-client relationship. The rules include (1) veracity or truth-telling; (2) confidentiality and privacy; and (3) fidelity (Beauchamp & Childress, 1989; Downie & Calman, 1987).

Respect for Autonomy

A basic assumption of moral philosophy is the inherent autonomy of each individual. Autonomy refers to the individual's personal self-determination and ability to act, free from controlling interference by others and from personal limitations. The concept of personal autonomy presumes the right and ability to make one's own voluntary, intentional choices, to maintain bodily integrity, and to live according to one's religion and beliefs (Wetle, 1987). It assumes that a person acts freely, not under duress. It also assumes that the individual's actions are not unduly constrained by the available choices, by his/her own weaknesses or limitations, or by the wishes of others.

Autonomy, thus, relates to individuals (the autonomous person) and to behaviors (autonomous actions). An autonomous person is someone who is 'competent' and 'of sound mind,' who, as a result, is able to make his/her own choices, to consent to, or reject 'care,' and to act in ways supported by his/her own desires, beliefs, plans, and preferences. Autonomous actions are those behaviors and acts that are intentionally taken by an individual, given the available information, the individual's understanding of the situation, and his/her own beliefs and desires, and that are taken without undue external influences or restrictions on options.

Professionals and others show respect for autonomy when, through their behavior, they take account of that person's own desires, feelings, and reasons and right to choose and decide for themselves. Professionals also respect the autonomy of others by providing individuals with any information available to them (the professional), that is needed to enable the client to make an informed decision, whereby his/her intentions and desires are supported. Respect is shown through the use of skill, shared wisdom, and support for the individual in making what are often very difficult choices.

Beneficence

While individuals are autonomous, there are many times when, due to human vulnerabilities and/or situational factors, the individual is not able to take the desired actions or achieve the desired ends. At such times it is morally appropriate (good, right) to act in such a way as to benefit the other person. These actions may prevent harm, remove harm, or actively promote good. Downie and Calman (1987) note that in the health and social care professions this behavior might more appropriately be referred to as "compassion," a combination of "emotion, positive help, and imaginative understanding," tempered with respect for the dignity of the individual (p. 55).

The moral requirements of compassion may be constrained. On the one hand, one's own beliefs and values about what is in the best interests of another person may be in conflict with that person's beliefs and values and, consequently, with their autonomy. In addition, beneficence in health and social care is constrained by the limitations on social resources available to provide help. Beneficence by professionals is a 'moral obligation,' to help another when certain conditions are met: Only when the helper (A) is aware of the relevant facts that helpee (B) is at risk of significant harm or loss, and that A's action is needed to prevent that harm, with a high probability of preventing or minimizing it, and that A's action would not create significant risks or harm for A, or that the benefit to B outweighs any burden or harm to A (Beauchamp & Childress, 1989).

Conflicts often arise between the moral principles of beneficence and autonomy in long-term care services. To some extent professional codes of ethics have put primary emphasis on the morality and necessity of beneficence, often to the neglect of individual autonomy. Physicians and others are taught to promote the 'best interests of the client.' However, the tendency is to define 'best interest' according to the professional judgment, knowledge and values, and in regard to the specific domain for which the professional provides care, e.g., health. Clients have a wider range of human values and concerns, such that their independent judgment about their needs or best interests differs from the needs or interests as defined more narrowly from the professional's framework.

Professionals, acting out of their commitment to beneficence, may make related decisions about disclosure and consent based on their medical care values, failing to recognize that the individual and not the professional is the 'pivotal decision-maker' (Beauchamp & Childress, 1989). Paternalism involves an individual, often a professional, taking actions that he/she deems to be in the best interest of the other (e.g., client), rather than letting the client make those choices or judgments. The underlying assumption of the professional is that he/she has superior knowledge and insight with regard to the potential harms or benefits. If the client disagrees or questions the decisions made, professionals may assume that the individual is not 'competent' to make a reasoned, informed choice, i.e., is not able to act autonomously.

Non-Maleficence

Related to the concepts of beneficence or compassion is that of non-maleficence, which suggests that individuals (i.e., professionals) have an obligation not to inflict harm or injury to others (Beauchamp & Childress, 1989). Harm can be defined to include actions that injure, disable, kill another person or those that undermine another's reputation, property, privacy, or liberty.

The obligation not to cause harm encompasses acts of 'commission' (actual actions taken) and acts of 'omission' (failing to take necessary action). Ethicists refer to a standard of due care, suggesting that carelessness and/or negligence may cause harm to others. To achieve the appropriate standard of care, professionals should have proper training, skills, and diligence, and should adhere to professional standards of practice. If that is done, then mistakes which inevitably occur cannot be considered to be negligence. Even if it is easier to do things for persons than to let them do for themselves, impairing a person's ability to make an informed choice is considered to be a form of harm. Pity, with its passive sympathy and element of condescension, also can harm the dignity of another (Downie & Calman, 1987).

Non-maleficence also underlies certain arguments that raise the issue of the "slippery slope," typically used to question the morality of mercy killing or passive euthanasia. As Beauchamp and Childress (1989) note, these arguments force us to examine "whether unacceptable harms may result from attractive and apparently innocent first steps" (p. 139). The overriding thread in the moral fabric of society is 'respect for human life,' so ethicists argue that any steps which remove barriers to killing may unravel the moral fabric.

However, in the same vein, the termination of treatment which has proven ineffective should not typically be considered harmful. The moral stance with regard to treatment falls into three categories: those treatments which are obligatory (or right), which offer a reasonable hope of benefit without excessive expense, pain or inconvenience; nonobligatory treatment, where the expense, pain, and/or inconvenience outweigh potential benefits, if any. Finally, treatments which are clearly not in the client's best interests are wrong; this may be pointless treatment which cannot offer a benefit, or where the burden or harm caused far outweigh benefits (Beauchamp & Childress, 1989).

Justice

This moral concept suggests that the distribution of the benefits and burdens of society should be done "fairly," according to what a person 'deserves' or 'what is due them.' "Injustice arises when one is denied that to which one is entitled" (Beauchamp & Childress, 1989, p. 257). Distributive justice is the attempt to ensure that there is a correct distribution of social benefits and burdens within society, based on relevant qualities or characteristics of persons or groups. Typically, it addresses how scarce resources are distributed among competing parties and how costs are distributed, as well. Alternative risks and benefits of various distribution strategies must be weighed, considering both who should get the benefits and who should bear the costs or risks. Professionals in the long-term care field deal with these issues on a daily basis, given the limited public resources for health and social services. From the professional's perspective the principle of justice is supported when one can 'treat people equally or fairly,' by 'treating like cases alike.' Given the complexity of situations and factors that impact on individuals served in long-term care, however, it is a continuing challenge to professionals in the field to establish relevant criteria of "likeness," as well as strategies for allocating both benefits and costs.

ETHICAL RULES FOR PROFESSIONAL-CLIENT RELATIONSHIPS

Rules Governing Professional-Client Relationship

Derived from the above moral and ethical concepts are broad sets of rules that should govern professional-client relationships. Beauchamp and Childress (1989) refer to these as rules of veracity, privacy, confidentiality, and fidelity.

Veracity

Veracity is the obligation to tell the truth and not to lie or deceive a client. Few of the codes of professional ethics explicitly require the professional to "tell the truth." In many instances, in the health care field particularly, the decision to "tell the truth" or "not to deceive the client" is one for which the professional may use "professional judgment." Ethical principles suggest that if a professional is to really respect the autonomy of a client, they must tell the truth to the client, so that the individual can make an 'informed' decision or choice. If a client discovers that a professional has lied or withheld the truth from him/her, it may undermine the "trust" that is central to a positive client-professional relationship, and may further undermine the willingness of the client to agree to and/or comply with the plan of treatment recommended by the professional.

Privacy and Confidentiality

These are intertwined, yet distinct rules for the professional-client relationship. Privacy refers to the client's right and ability to limit "access" by others to personal matters and/or one's own person, including the body and all its parts, as well as intimate relationships. Confidentiality refers to the moral behavior of a professional who has access to private, intimate information about another. Basically it assumes that such information or knowledge is still private, and that access to such information is shared with others only with the client's consent. Clients should be informed by professionals about their rights to continued privacy, as well as their own personal right to access any information in their records, and their rights to control access to such records and information (Beauchamp & Childress, 1989).

Fidelity

Fidelity is the implicit contract between the professional and the client that the client's welfare is what is being promoted by the actions and treatments offered by the professional. Further, fidelity is a commitment to remain faithful and diligent in promoting the client's well-being, keeping promises made, and not making promises that cannot be kept. It is the moral commitment not to neglect or abandon the client.

ARTICULATING MORAL ARGUMENTS AND THOUGHTS

As previously noted by Abramson (1985), to have an effective ethics committee, members of that group must become familiar and skilled with evaluating and expressing logical moral arguments. Abrams (1993) suggests that an ethics committee can serve as an "Ideal Ethical Observer" (i.e., omniscient, omnipercipient, disinterested, dispassionate, and consistent) if the participants learn to avoid adversarial behavior and acknowledge that "ethical principles are not pathways which lead to answers. Rather they are borders and boundaries within which reasonable alternatives can be gathered" (p. 2).

Downie and Calman (1987) note that participants must understand the nature of logical arguments, that is, that they involve premises or assumptions (which may be either true or false) and conclusions (which may be true or false and may also follow from the premises or not). Premises which do not support the conclusions which follow are invalid arguments, and if conclusions are to be true, then the premises must be true.

There are many fallacies that arise under the guise of moral arguments. Particularly problematic are errors in fact, opinions stated as facts, unstated assumptions of moral rules or facts, conflicts between moral principles, and ambiguities in words and knowledge (Downie and Calman, 1987). One fallacy common among professionals is the assumption that professional values should prevail in certain domains, such as physicians in the realm of physical health and pathologies, clergy for spiritual, and attorneys for legal and contractual domains (Abrams, 1993). In this regard, many professionals tend to argue from their own value system rather than the broader societal set of ethical principles.

As with any new vocabulary and concepts, individuals need to spend time discussing the concepts and using the vocabulary to reach a level of competency and comfort, and must learn to recognize errors in their logic and application of terms. Group members must work with these concepts to achieve a sense of ease with the basic moral concepts and with assessing and expressing moral arguments. They must become accustomed to stating their own assumptions and premises more explicitly, having the logic of their arguments questioned in a non-threatening manner, and, consequently, expressing and examining their own arguments and conclusions. If all members of the group can achieve a level of ease in assessing and expressing moral arguments, the group or committee can become a safe and much-needed forum for expressing and exploring the moral and ethical conflicts faced by professionals within the long-term care continuum.

As quoted by Gibson and Kushner (1986), one hospital ethics

committee expressed the goals of this process well: " . . . A movement away from a private, idiosyncratic approach in which my reasons and rationale must satisfy my personal integrity; toward an approach in which reasons, rationales, and meanings, and evaluations are subject to reflection of others with common concerns. Ethical discernment moves from the realm of private judgment to the arena of discourse and communal review" (p. 11).

CLARIFYING AND PRIORITIZING ETHICAL PRINCIPLES AND VALUES

Once an ethics committee has developed a basic level of shared understanding of ethical concepts and meanings, members can begin to identify the most pressing ethical issues within the segment of the long-term care continuum to which they will act as advisor. Collopy (1991) suggests that professional caregivers often must balance or prioritize four different kinds of ethical responsibilities in the delivery of long-term care: (1) the responsibility to provide clients with appropriate care; (2) the responsibility to respect and support the role of informal caregivers; (3) the responsibility for public accountability to conduct themselves according to professional standards of good practice; and (4) the responsibility to equitably distribute scarce resources.

In the committee's self-education process, members may discover that they value or prioritize these various ethical responsibilities differently. They may also discover other kinds of ethical concerns that play a role within the service system to which they act as advisor. The ethics committee may begin to discuss actual cases, in order to sort out these different values and priorities and to establish a hierarchy of values and responsibilities appropriate to their care system.

However, as Abrams (1993) notes, "value issues cannot be answered by authority" (p. 3). It is important that both individual and societal issues be considered and weighed. Since most ethics committees are not decision-making bodies, the "ideal ethics committee" will involve a societal "microcosm," that can provide the system's decision-makers with a broad range of feelings, knowledge, values and perspectives through an objective review of actual case situations (Abrams, 1993). Differences of perspectives add value to the committee, rather than diminishing its worth. Working first with "case studies" (after the fact situations) and then with actual, ongoing cases will enable the group to develop proficiency in discussing the difficult, value-laded matters in an objective way.

Gibson & Kushner (1986) note that self-education is a continuing process for an ethics committee. The committee members are constantly learning and reassessing values and priorities. Once the committee or group has completed an initial period of self-education, it becomes important that the committee (a relatively small group of professionals in the system) provide education to others within the institutional or community care setting, to include decision-makers, staff, and clients and family members. The committee will need to be able to communicate clearly about the nature of the ethical concerns, values and priorities, that play a role in the long-term care service system. The committee can also become a source of advice and guidance about how individual professionals, service teams, agencies, and the entire care system can apply ethical principles in their delivery of care.

LOGISTICS WITHIN THE ETHICS COMMITTEE

As previously noted, if an ethics committee is to be effective there must be a mission statement for the group, and a plan that spells out the goals and purposes of the group and its role and placement within the care setting. Typical goals for an ethics committee include education, policy advice, and case consultation within the specific care setting (AARP, 1990).

Getting the right participants on an ethics committee is an important logistical detail, according to some. In the American Association of Homes for the Aged and American Association of Retired Persons joint guidelines, it is recommended to have a committee small enough to be manageable, and yet large enough to encompass diverse points of view and to function with members absent. Ideally, the committee should reflect a multi-disciplinary membership, representative of those which must interact within the caregiving context and when specific cases are under consideration, with specialties or disciplines appropriate to the issue under discussion. Another

desirable quality of individual members, is persons who are reflec-
tive, open and cooperative, rather than fast acting and noncoopera-
tive (AARP, 1990). Abrams (1993) notes that one goal of the ethics
committee that functions as an advisory board is to emulate the
"ideal ethical observer" described in the medical ethics literature.
Such an observer should be omniscient, omnipercipient, disinterested and impartial, dispassionate, and consistent, qualities rarely
found in individual humans. Thus, he suggests that ethics committees should have a "broad-based, multi-disciplinary" membership,
where a "multiplicity of values can be represented and offered to
the primary decision-maker"(p. 3). This will be an effort to accurately represent the diversity of society, and the reality that society
has values related to limits and acceptable choices.

An effective ethics committee will identify and collect resources
that facilitate members' self-education efforts. These resources include persons with expertise related to ethics, as well as articles and
books dealing with ethical principles in long-term care and health
and social care settings and case-studies that enable the group to
explore the ethical and moral concepts.

Finally, to be effective, the committee must establish a protocol
(standards and procedures) for its actions in reviewing, discussing
and giving advice about specific cases. Ensuring a common understanding of the mission and purpose among all members is critical.
From that point procedures related to calling meetings, setting
agendas, record keeping, discussion procedures, and the development of educational materials or sessions, and policy recommenda-
tions all need to be clarified. Frequency of meetings, essential or
core membership for a meeting, issues of confidentiality, how to
respond to urgent situations, and similar matters can be carefully
delineated. With a clear protocol, the group can ensure that persons
bringing cases to the group for consultation bring the key types of
information essential for the group to effectively review the situation. A good protocol also serves to focus group discussion on the
ethical issues, thereby diminishing the likelihood of irrelevant issues being introduced. The protocol also gives each person the right
and responsibility to express feelings and perspectives, to direct
such comments to the case under review, and not to direct hostile
comments and accusations at others within the group.

CONCLUSION

Long-term care services both in nursing homes and community-based care settings have a wide array of health, social, and resource elements that pose ethical dilemmas in the delivery of care. The adoption of an ethics committee model of care can be used to illuminate and clarify some of these issues. Such committees or discussions should not be reserved for acute care settings, as issues of ethical action occur every day in the delivery of long-term care services in the clients' homes, in care coordination settings, and in the nursing home. Such a committee can enhance professional functioning, by reducing stress and providing a sounding board to review decisions and choices that trouble the professional. They can improve inter-professional collaboration, by increasing understanding of the differences in values and priorities among different professions. Understanding may not lead to agreement, but it can reduce the sense of surprise, even shock, that may occur when professional values and priorities collide. Further, the ethics committee can help enhance the ethical quality of intra- and inter-institutional decisions and actions.

REFERENCES

Abrams, F. R. (1993). The ideal ethics committee as the "ideal ethical observer." In Denver Community Bioethics Committee, *Manual of Policies, Procedures, and Resources*. Unpublished manuscript.

Abramson, Marcia. (1985). Caught in the middle. *Generations. X*, 35-37.

American Association of Retired Persons (AARP). (1990). *Ethics committees: Allies in long-term care–A guidebook to forming an ethics committee*. A joint project of the American Association of Homes for the Aging and American Association of Retired Persons.

Beauchamp, T. L. & Childress, J. F. (1989). *Principles of biomedical ethics, 3rd edition*. New York: Oxford University Press.

Collopy, B. J. (1991, May). *Ethical issues in community-based long term care*. Paper presented at the National Council on the Aging Annual Meeting. Miami Beach.

Denver Community Bioethics Committee. (1993, January). *Manual of Policies, Procedures, and Resources*. Unpublished manuscript.

Downie, R. S. & Calman, L. C. (1987). *Healthy respect: Ethics in health care*. Boston: Faber & Faber.

Gibson, J. M & Kushner, T. K. (1986). Ethics committees: How are they doing?
    Hastings Center Report, 16, 9-11.
Wetle, T. T. (1987). Ethical aspects of decision-making for and with the elderly. In
    M. B. Kapp, H. E. Pies, Jr. & A. E. Doudera (Eds.). *Legal and ethical aspects
    of health care for the elderly.* Pp. 258-267. Ann Arbor, MI: Health Administra-
    tion Press.

APPENDIX

CASE ILLUSTRATIONS OF ETHICAL DILEMMAS FROM LONG TERM CARE SETTINGS

The following case studies are included here to illustrate typical ethical
dilemmas and issues that have been faced in settings across the long-term
care continuum in one mid-sized Western city. Each case study highlights
some of the ethical issues the professionals involved in such settings may
confront. It is our hope that these case studies may benefit the group that is
still struggling with ethical concepts and seeking to prioritize values and
ethical responsibilities, before they move to considering actual case consultation in their own service system.

Case Study #1–Nursing Home Setting

Of particular concern in nursing homes are issues of resident rights. An
increased awareness of these rights is in part due to federal and state
regulations which make them a priority ethical concern. Residents, family
members and others may question recommended medical treatments and,
at times, may refuse medical intervention altogether. With the passage of
the Patient Self-Determination Act, adults are asserting greater control
over their own health care. The following case illustrates some of the
ethical issues facing professionals in the nursing home context.

Mr. Smith entered the nursing home because he had a stroke and his
sister could no longer care for him in her home. Mr. Smith, from the day of
his arrival at the nursing home displayed very little interest in interacting
with the other residents. He was frequently gruff and difficult to get along
with. However, neither the staff nor his family members ever considered
him to be incompetent.

Recently, due to the side effects of his stroke and his choice not to
comply with a physician's recommended medical treatment for his dia-

betes (keeping his legs elevated and managing his diet), Mr. Smith experienced blood flow problems in his leg. Subsequently, the physician indicated to the client that his leg would have to be amputated, since the blood flow was so impaired that the leg would develop gangrene, which would be both extremely painful and deadly. The client refused to undergo the amputation, clearly stating to the staff and the physician that he would "just take his chances." The staff, in an effort to make sure that the client fully understood the ramifications of his decision, reviewed with him again what his medical condition was and what would happen if the leg was not amputated. The client remained adamant about his decision at that time.

The facility staff, concerned that their own values and preferences were clouding the issues, requested the assistance of the local ombudsman. The ombudsman attempted to determine if the client was an autonomous person, based on information obtained from the client, his family, the staff, and the physician. She deemed that, even though the client was responding to his health problems in a highly emotional manner, the client was competent and could not be denied his right to refuse treatment. She also attempted to obtain, in a confidential manner, other opinions regarding the intensity and extent of pain the client could be expected to suffer, since this seemed to be a key issue for the physician and other professional staff. While all the medical professionals consulted agreed that gangrene, once developed, would poison the client's system, resulting in death, the speed of the process and the level of pain he was likely to experience were variable.

The facility staff, along with the Ombudsman, then met with the family and the physician to discuss the case further. The client was also invited to attend the meeting, but refused. In the meeting the physician expressed his conviction that the client must be incompetent, since he was refusing the amputation (the physician had never questioned the client's competence when he was relatively compliant). During the conference the family and the facility staff both clearly stated that they were not happy with the decision of the client *not* to have the amputation. However, neither the family nor the staff felt that the client was incompetent.

At this conference it was decided that the facility staff would continue to educate the client about the progression of the gangrene, to ensure that he was fully informed regarding his medical condition and prognosis. The physician stood firm in this belief that the client was incompetent. He also stated that he felt it was the client's moral obligation to society to have his leg amputated, because of the discomfort that the odor of his rotting flesh would cause for other residents living in the nursing home.

Shortly after the case conference adult protection was called in and a competency hearing was set up. At the preliminary hearing it was determined that the client *was* competent. However, shortly thereafter the client changed his mind and had his leg amputated, either because the pain had become too great or he had decided that he wanted to live.

Discussion Issues for an Ethics Committee–Case 1

While the resident asserted that he did not want the prescribed medical intervention in the early stages of this situation, the ethics committee might wish to grapple with the following questions:

- Did the resident truly understand the consequences of his choice?
- Was he truly making an autonomous choice (i.e., was he able to understand the possible outcome of his choice, was he really stating a choice, or was he simply trying to come to terms with two courses of action, both of which were personally unacceptable?)
- When professionals deem that a choice that a client is making is clearly *not in his own best interests*, should they take actions that will be in the client's best interests (beneficence vs. paternalism)?
- Was permitting the client his choice to refuse treatment harmful to others, and would such harm outweigh the benefit to the client of exercising an autonomous choice?
- When a patient acts in his *own best interests,* but his choice is viewed to require professionals to fail to exercise "due care," how does their right to autonomy and choice enter in . . . can they refuse to permit the client to remain in the facility, or can individual professionals refuse to provide care?
- Is it appropriate for professionals to decide that *incompetence* is self-evident when a client refuses to *comply* with a recommended course of treatment, even if failure to comply is life-threatening?
- To what extent did the physician and staff break the moral rules of *veracity* by painting the "worst case scenario" for this client?
- Is *justice* served by urging someone who does not want service to accept services?
- Is it appropriate to provide "treatment" when the prognosis for survival is limited, even with the prescribed treatment?

Case Study #2–Case Management Program

Community based programs such as case management agencies are frequently expected to deal effectively with very difficult situations. Clients who may no longer have the ability to adequately take care of themselves due to cognitive or physical limitations, may insist on remaining in their own homes. Many times there are no family members to provide support or assistance, or those family members who are available are disinterested, or are totally frustrated with the older family member's choices or decisions. The following situation represents one such situation, which raised many ethical and moral concerns for the case managers and their cooperating provider agencies.

An elderly Hispanic woman, Mrs. Soto, requested case management assistance to enable her to receive home care services. An insulin-dependent diabetic, confined to a wheelchair for mobility due to the severity of her diabetes, she was physically but not cognitively impaired. After a few home visits, the case manager found the client to be uncooperative. Mrs. Soto was frequently not home when service providers arrived, even though the appointments had been agreed to with the case manager. Both the case manager and the provider agency staff reminded Mrs. Soto to notify them if she could not keep her appointments, and then they could reschedule her home visits. At times when Mrs. Soto was served at home, agency staff observed that she did not take her medication in a timely manner, and was not observing the physician-prescribed diet.

As a result of her non-compliance her health failed and she was admitted to the local hospital. At the end of her hospital stay, the hospital social worker (discharge planner) contacted the case management agency to facilitate Mrs. Soto's return to her own home, with in-home services. The case manager informed the social worker that the client could not qualify for the case management program because all the home health care agencies refused to serve her, given her history of noncompliance. The client did return to her home in the community anyway, but had to rely solely on her family for assistance.

Discussion Issues for an Ethics Committee–Case 2

A community-service/case management ethics committee could have assisted the agencies involved in resolving several ethical questions and/or issues:

- Were the case management and home health professionals justified in refusing to serve the client? Had the client been provided with sufficient information to understand the possible consequence of her prior behavior (missing scheduled appointments)?
- Were the staff exercising "due care" with regard to this client?

- Do staff frustrations with clients who do not "comply" with the prescribed treatment, that professionals view as being "in the best interests" of the client, justify a refusal to offer services (beneficence)?
- To what extent had the client been consulted regarding the original plan of treatment (offered choices), and, if not consulted, was the refusal to comply with treatment this client's way of communicating her preferences?
- Since most human service agencies have extremely limited budgets, is it *just* to continue to attempt to serve a client who is not cooperative and who does not follow the recommended treatment?
- Was the agencies' refusal to serve this client at the time of discharge, an indication of a lack of *fidelity* on their part to this client?

Case Study # 3–Home Health Care

Med-Health Home Health Care was providing services to two elderly sisters, Ethel and Martha Jones. The sisters had lived together for many years and had no other living relatives except for and even older sister, who lived in a nursing home in another state. The home health care agency staff became increasingly concerned, as they observed the sisters becoming more physically and cognitively impaired. Ethel and Martha both stated that they would like to stay in their home. They felt that with the regular assistance of the home health agency staff they would get along just fine. Either they did not want to admit their increasing disabilities, or they were unaware of the changes in their condition.

Med-Health continued to provide in-home services to both sisters until Martha fell, was sent to the hospital, and then, upon discharge, was moved to a nursing home. After several months in the nursing home Martha convinced her doctor to discharge her back to her own home. Although the home health care agency staff agreed to start-up services for Martha again, they were not feeling very comfortable with the situation. Martha stayed at home for only a few months, then she returned to a nursing home.

Med-Health staff continued to have concerns about Ethel. They found her becoming more forgetful and confused. She was unable to remember to take her medication, prepare food, manage her own finances, and so on. Med-Health staff decided to contact the Adult Protection regarding her situation. An Adult Protection worker did speak with Ethel, although it was not clear how much time was spent on this case, and what type of investigation was conducted. According to the Adult Protection worker, Ethel appeared to be competent, and so the adult protection case was closed. This lack of cooperation by the Adult Protection unit led the

Med-Health staff to become quite frustrated, as they felt that Ethel was at high-risk, unable to make sound decisions, and that the agency was no longer able to adequately meet her needs. However, the staff also felt that stopping services to Ethel would be life-threatening.

Prior to the development of her confusion, Ethel had indicated to Med-Health that she and her sister were financially secure. Their monthly income was sufficient to pay for their living expenses and the services they were receiving from the agency. After Ethel appeared no longer able to manger her own financial matters, the Med-Health social worker assisted her in checking on saving accounts. However, the worker and the agency were uncomfortable with this role. As a provider of services, they did not feel that this was an appropriate role for them to play. However, since there were no other agencies willing to assist Ethel with her finances, they saw no other choice, if they were to pursue the "best interests" of the client.

Ethel eventually decided that she would move to a personal care boarding home, which would permit her to keep her small dog. Med-Health staff were pleased that Ethel was acknowledging her need for another living arrangement. However, they again felt that it was not their role to help her select a home, or to make her financial arrangements for care. At this time they again recontacted the Department of Social Services, to seek assistance for Ethel in these endeavors.

Discussion Issues for an Ethics Committee–Case 3

As with many other agencies who provide services to the elderly in their homes, Med-Health staff found themselves involved in aspects of care which they were not able or willing to provide. In this case they found that they were becoming involved in many aspects of the client's life. When they saw that the client's needs were going to be long-term they sought outside assistance. This agency could have benefited from a community-based ethics committee to explore many dimensions of this situation. Questions that the staff grappled with included:

- How to deal with a long-term client (fidelity) when her behavior indicated that she was no longer competent to act in her own best interests (i.e., autonomously)?
- How to define an appropriate role where the agency is able to exercise due care, without compromising the privacy and confidentiality of the relationship?
- What to do in situations where there was no one other than the client to act in her own behalf, at a time when she has shown limited competence?

- Is the agency guilty of doing harm through omission, if they don't provide services the client clearly needs?
- How long and in what situation can a professional indicate that the demands of the situation exceed their ability/willingness to provide care?
- To what extent is the agency guilty of nonmaleficence, if providing assistance in financial matters, where they may have a conflict of interest, since they charge her for their services?

Ethics and Values in Music Therapy for Persons Who Are Elderly

Alicia Ann Clair

Through a review of the literature, ethics refer to morals, morality and rules of conduct. Further defined, ethics relate to moral action, motive or character, particularly right and wrong. Ethical considerations in music therapy practice with persons who are elderly, therefore, refer to the right and wrong of practice using music as a medium of therapeutic intervention.

Ethics are influenced by values, and the values of each music therapist are well integrated into therapeutic processes. It is essential, then, that music therapists, as well as other helping professionals, be aware of their personal values and the influence these values have on their professional practices.

Music therapy, as any other helping discipline, is focused on the development or maintenance of life quality for those who receive it. Quality of life, as defined by the medical profession, refers to the restoration of health, relief of pain and symptoms, and support of compromised function. It has grown out of a 15th century medical maxim which reads, "cure occasionally, relieve frequently, comfort always" (Jonsen, Siegler, & Winslade, 1982, p. 109). While music therapists do not claim to cure, they use music to provide relief, to

Alicia Ann Clair, PhD, Registered Music Therapist-Board Certified, is Professor and Director of Music Therapy, University of KS, Lawrence, KS, and Research Associate at the Veterans Affairs Medical Center in Topeka.

[Haworth co-indexing entry note]: "Ethics and Values in Music Therapy for Persons Who Are Elderly." Clair, Alicia Ann. Co-published simultaneously in *Activities, Adaptation & Aging* (The Haworth Press, Inc.) Vol. 18, No. 3/4, 1994, pp. 27-46; and: *Ethics and Values in Long Term Health Care* (ed: Patricia J. Villani) The Haworth Press, Inc., 1994, pp. 27-46. Multiple copies of this article/chapter may be purchased from The Haworth Document Delivery Center [1-800-3-HAWORTH; 9:00 a.m. - 5:00 p.m. (EST)].

support functional behaviors and, most assuredly, to comfort. Guided by a professional Code of Ethics (National Association for Music Therapy, 1987) and Standards of Clinical Practice (National Association for Music Therapy, 1987) they do this in a therapeutic context which may include the amelioration of physical discomforts and management of stressors to promote wellness, but also it may include delivering services which influence the psychological, social, and spiritual well-being of persons who are elderly.

There are ethical problems when considering the quality of life for any person. These stem from a placement of value on some feature of the human experience. Jonsen et al. (1982) indicate this value is subjective and is usually conceptualized by someone other than the one who is living the life. They go on to say that quality of life is based on facts which are defined or measured clinically, and are not based on the individual's preferences about the facts (p. 110). It would seem, then, that quality of life, and a sense of well-being associated with it, must certainly be decided by the one who lives the life, and not by an observer. Consequently, each individual must decide about his or her life quality, whether it is acceptable as it is or whether there is a desire for change. That decision hinges not only on the physical condition of the individual, but also on the social, psychological, and spiritual conditions as well.

QUALIFICATIONS OF A MUSIC THERAPIST

Anyone who provides music therapy services must have credentials which indicate their qualifications to do so. Included in these credentials is graduation from a music therapy academic program accredited at either the undergraduate or master's degree level by the American Association for Music Therapy or the National Association for Music Therapy. These accredited academic programs provide the theoretical constructs, research based knowledge, and clinical practice skill development necessary for a beginning professional. In addition, they provide a working knowledge of ethics as an entry level skill (Moranto, & Wheeler, 1986).

Following graduation, music therapists are certified through a national board examination which assures that they have at least entry level knowledge and skills to provide music therapy services.

After initial certification, music therapists are expected to maintain their board certification status through continuing education.

Music therapists who meet the contingencies for board certification have a thorough understanding of music therapy constructs and their applications to clinical practice. Early in their careers, these music therapists are most often general practitioners, and these therapists may develop specialty areas as they practice. One of these specialty areas is music therapy for persons who are elderly. Within this are subspecialties including music therapy for persons who are well and elderly, who are frail, who have dementia, and who are family members and/or caregivers for those who are old.

Whatever their practice specialty, music therapists must know and indicate clearly their knowledge, skills, and abilities to deliver services. They have the responsibility to refuse services to those who request that which goes beyond their competencies. They may, however, make referrals to other music therapists who have the background and experience to provide such services. Once services are initiated, the music therapists have the responsibility to stay within the boundaries of their competencies to provide them.

Professional boundaries are also an issue when determining whether or not there is enough time allowed for services to affect change and whether there is appropriate follow-up to those services. Follow-up can be critical when persons are involved in short-term programs where personal responses may not have time for closure or resolution. This is particularly important where such programs are conducted in groups, and it is not possible for individuals to communicate with the music therapist. In this circumstance, the therapist has a grave responsibility to leave issues closed for which there can be no solution or resolution due to time constraints, or personal limitations of the music therapist or the participant. Before any attempt is made to provide services in music therapy, there must be a careful assessment of an individual's needs and the capacity of the music therapist to meet them in the time allotted. If it is not possible for the music therapy program to be efficacious for the individual in the time allowed, then the program should not be offered.

Of particular concern are those persons who do not have the credentials to practice as music therapists, but who claim to deliver therapeutic services with music. These persons may or may not have an adequate awareness of the power of music to influence physiological, social, and psychological responses in individuals. If they are aware of such influences, they are not trained to assess individual's needs, or to design, implement, and evaluate programming specific to those needs. These practitioners may have successes with music, because music is a remarkable medium, indeed. These successes, however, may not meet the Standards for Clinical Practice (National Association for Music Therapy, 1987), and/or they may not be as efficacious as those that are facilitated by a qualified music therapist who is board certified.

MUSIC THERAPY PROGRAM INVOLVEMENT

Any music therapy program is predicated on the assessment of individual client's needs, and ongoing interventions are adjusted or maintained through careful evaluation of individual client's responses. While programs can be implemented in groups or in one-to-one situations, program involvement for each individual is contingent upon each person's commitment to the therapeutic process.

Persons who are well and elderly may or may not have an interest in music therapy due to their receptivity to therapeutic interventions in general. Attitudes may vary from those who do not want music therapy because they have no apparent illness, and consequently they perceive no need for intervention, to those who desire an intervention to manage stress, add to life interests, and enhance wellness. For those who are interested and receptive to music therapy, though they are well, strategies may include stress management, personal enrichment through imagery and music, development of music skills, and spiritual growth, among others.

Persons who are elderly and have become physically frail, or have intellectual frailties due to conditions which result in deterioration of their cognitive abilities, may find music therapy interventions helpful in maintaining their social, psychological, and physical functions. These interventions are designed to promote independence in appropriate functional areas for as long as possible, and may be implemented in the home, senior centers, day care and respite care centers and in residential care facilities. Music therapy interventions can be adjusted to allow for individual differences and changes in functionality while it is used for such purposes as stress management, relief from physical discomfort, fear, and/or anxiety, physical rehabilitation through motor integration and exercise adherence, social integration and relief from isolation, emotional expression and communication, control over the environment, reality orientation and validation, reminiscence and life review, spiritual growth and support, sensory stimulation, and enhancement of life in a time of loss.

In addition to providing programs for those who are old, music therapy interventions can also be designed for family members and/or caregivers to provide stress relief and management, opportunities for personal enrichment, and opportunities to interact purposefully and meaningfully with care receivers. With this interaction comes the restoration of emotional intimacy so essential to satisfactory relationships.

The most important consideration in music therapy program design, implementation, and continuation is the welfare of the individual client who must have the most efficacious intervention possible. When the individual can no longer benefit from the intervention, it is essential to terminate it. At this point, the music therapist may make a referral to another therapist, or may advise the individual that further intervention is unwarranted. The music therapist must also terminate therapeutic relationships, or avoid establishing them in the first place, when those relationships are likely to interfere with the therapist's professional judgment or objectivity, i.e., in the case of providing intervention for a family member or a personal friend (National Association of Music Therapy, Code of Ethics, 1987).

Music Therapist and Client Relationship

The basis of the relationship between the individual and the music therapist is the therapist's unconditional acceptance of and respect for the individual as a person. This acceptance and respect fosters decision making at whatever levels the individual can function physically, socially, emotionally, spiritually, and psychologically. This functionality is then supported and encouraged through the therapist's knowledge, skills, and abilities of the therapeutic applications of music and is influenced as little as possible by the cultural, emotional, and intellectual biases of the music therapist. With this focus on enhancement of functional strengths, the music therapist designs and implements programming which compliments the individual's cultural background, and sustains the individual's integrity and dignity as a person. Such programming avoids involving individuals in programs which require responses that are discordant with their values and beliefs, e.g., requiring a person to dance who has believed for a lifetime that dancing is a grave sin, using mental images that an individual thinks are evil influences, using Christian religious music with someone who is non-Christian, or using popular music of the 1890's with some one who was born in 1920, to name a few. While any of these uses of music might be incorporated with the best intentions, they can have deleterious effects, some of which can be quite serious.

Within the relationship between the individual and the music therapist is the issue of confidentiality. To protect confidentiality for individuals, the music therapist must not disclose information regarding their behaviors outside the group of professionals who provide direct care to them. In exception, music therapists, and all helping professionals, have a responsibility to protect those who are likely to injure themselves or others, and to protect a potential victim from the client's violent behavior (Corey, Corey, & Callanan, 1988). Music therapists must know the laws concerning confidentiality and the right to privacy in the states in which they practice, and they must act accordingly.

VALUES IN MUSIC THERAPY

Values are the basis for the relationships between clients who are elderly and music therapists who work with them. Ultimately, the music therapist must value individuals who have become elderly to establish interventions that are most beneficial to them. If there is little interest or reverence for elders, the music therapist must pursue professional opportunities elsewhere.

The values of music therapists as people with cultural backgrounds, belief systems, and histories influence strongly their dealings with individual clients who are elderly. Even when music therapists are careful not to impose their values on others, those values can influence clients in subtle ways, e.g., when the music therapist attends to certain issues and not to others, or when nonverbal indications of approval and disapproval are given.

All music therapists must know their own values and know when they are opposed to those of a client. Then the therapist must be astutely aware of possibilities for subtle influences and exercise great care to avoid them; but, when the values between the music therapist and client clash to the point that a functional relationship cannot be developed or maintained, the music therapist must refer the client to another therapist.

Physical Functionality as a Value in Aging

One of the most highly valued abilities in persons who are elderly is physical function. Such function in maintained or rehabilitated through medical interventions and exercise, but exercise programs are difficult for persons with physical conditions that lead to discomfort when engaged in physical activity. Adherence to and endurance through exercise regimens, therefore, becomes an issue in rehabilitation and physical maintenance. Music therapists use music to distract from the discomfort and to motivate participation. In addition, new and impressive research findings indicate the powerful influence of music and rhythm on motor integration in physical rehabilitation for persons who have suffered strokes and other neurological impairments (Thaut, Schleiffers, & Davis, 1992; McIntosh, Thaut, Rice, & Prassas, 1993).

While music therapy may enhance and facilitate participation in exercise programs and physical therapy and while music remarkably influences motor integration, music therapists must collaborate with physical therapists and other appropriate health care professionals to design and implement physical rehabilitation interventions. Music therapists do not have the knowledge and skills to implement physical rehabilitation programs without input from appropriate health care professionals. Concomitantly, the expertise concerning music with exercise must come from the music therapist, who has the knowledge and training to design music strategies which best match and lead movement tempi in exercise regimens and otherwise facilitate rehabilitation.

With the value for physical flexibility comes the value for stress management in the maintenance and restoration of physical health. Most music therapists are trained to use relaxation techniques which are integrated with music to help individuals learn to manage stress which results from anxiety, fear, and physical discomfort or pain. These can be manifest in several ways including physical symptoms of hypertension or physical illness and disease, agitation, or combativeness.

Music therapists know that effectiveness of any stress management strategy with music depends on each client's preference for the music and his or her usual reactions to it. When individuals are nonverbal, or otherwise unable to communicate verbally their preferences, careful observations of their reactions to music will give clear indications of its' viability through facial expressions, body postures, and calmed or agitated reactions.

Music therapists also know that music which has effective stress management properties will be different for almost everyone. These individual differences preclude using music and relaxation approaches which are marketed for successful function to a broad audience. Without attention to individual preferences for and responses to music, effectiveness is lost.

Social Interaction and Engagement as a Value in Aging

Music therapy practice is often predicated on the fact that humans are social beings who are happiest and healthiest when they are with others (Gaston, 1968). The need for social intervention, therefore, arises when people have the desire to belong with others, but for some reason they are incapable of it. With persons who are elderly there may not be the opportunity because they have lived so long that they have lost family and friends through death. They may not know how to initiate new relationships or they may not be involved in the social structures where this might happen, e.g., church, senior center, or community organizations. On the other hand, they may have a progressive dementia, or another debilitating cognitive condition, which limits their social abilities to engage with others in meaningful and purposeful activities. They may also have physical limitations which make access to groups of people impossible.

Whatever the reason for social isolation and inactivity, music has the power to draw people together for a common purpose (Gaston, 1968). Through the expertise of the music therapist, these music experiences may be designed to attract persons of many age ranges and cultural backgrounds making it possible to form intergenerational groups, multigenerational groups, and groups of persons who share the same age cohort. These persons may be either diverse or similar in their cultural backgrounds, but they value meaningful, musical experiences where persons are mutually supportive and accepting, and where they can share feelings of belonging, along with a sense of feeling needed by others. The strategies used by the music therapist in these groups must incorporate the music preferences of all group members. In this context the music therapist is guided by knowledge, skills, and abilities to facilitate social viability with music, and not by personal desires or needs for recognition.

For nonverbal group members, the social interaction may occur only in the form of playing musical instruments, primarily rhythm instruments. While the persons have lost the skills to engage meaningfully with others, they may still value social integration. The structure of the rhythm during the music makes it possible even for those who are severely regressed in dementia to participate with others (Clair & Bernstein, 1990a; Clair & Bernstein, 1990b).

With instrumental playing, it is essential to use appropriate professional instruments. Toy instruments, or rhythm band instruments for children detract from the dignity of the individual and should never be used. In addition, kitchen implements incorporated into a "kitchen band" are silly and likewise undignified. The use of toys and kitchen implements heighten attention to the losses experienced in later years, and do not contribute to a strength based focus.

Psychological Values in Aging

While values are associated with many psychological functions in aging, several are currently particularly pertinent to music therapy practice. These include the values for reminiscence and life review, emotional expression, reality orientation and validation, music skill development and aesthetic experience as life enhancement.

Reminiscence and Life Review. Some professionals consider reminiscence and life review an essential component of satisfactory adjustment in aging (Wylie, 1990), but not all persons desire to reminisce about their lives. They may have little satisfaction with life and may have realized few, or none, of their dreams. As a result, they have no desire to focus their attention on their disappoint-ments, and they are particularly opposed to the attempts of others to bring memories of regret to their awareness. With such individuals, it is imperative to respect their preference to avoid reminiscence and life review activities.

When persons value reminiscence and choose to involve them-selves in it, the music therapist has a powerful medium to stimulate memories, evoke emotions, and bring to awareness other extramus-ical associations. These associations with music are very individu-alized, but persons in the same age cohort will likely share some commonalties through the events or times they all experienced. Certain songs can tap these common experiences and can therefore be used to stimulate discussion about them, e.g., "The White Cliffs of Dover" may be used to stimulate discussions of individual expe-riences during World War II.

Though the power of music to raise associations to awareness occur generally as planned, sometimes the unexpected happens. The music may evoke responses of anger, frustration, grief and other feelings that require resolution. Often these responses are not apparent until the music is used. In a therapeutic context, the music therapist can facilitate discussions of such associations, even when they are not anticipated. Those not trained in music therapy may not be aware that music can stimulate unexpected reactions such as these, and they may be ill-equipped to deal with them if they do.

Emotional Expressions. In addition to reminiscence and life re-view, music therapy can serve as a means for emotional expression. It must not be overlooked, however, that certain individuals are very emotionally expressive while others are threatened by emo-tions. The desire for expression and the openness to it are based in individual persons' histories. These histories are defined initially by cultural contexts and subsequently by communities and families within those cultures. Persons who indicate a need, or a preference, to remain private in their thoughts and feelings must be allowed to do so.

Individuals who chose emotional expression as part of their participation in music therapy must receive unconditional acceptance of the information they choose to share. These persons must also be allowed time to process this material with a music therapist trained to deal with emotional reactions. If the music therapist is relatively inexperienced and does not know how to facilitate resolution of feelings, or has any personal difficulty whatsoever concerning the emotional content of the session, then the situation which can stimulate such content must be avoided. Likewise, the music therapist has the responsibility to avoid stimulating emotional reactions in persons who are ill-equipped to deal with them, or for whom the material would be anxiety provoking or otherwise deleterious. This might include such things as avoiding discussions of past, painful experiences that the individual has removed from current awareness, e.g., the death of the individual's young child years earlier. To arouse emotions concerning this material would lead only to more suffering and misery. It is best left alone unless the individual expresses a desire to discuss it. At that time, music may be used to evoke memories and feelings, to embrace the feelings, to name them, to talk about them, and to finally let them go.

Even while exercising caution to stimulate emotional reactions in those who desire them and to avoid deleterious experiences, the music therapist is aware that music is a powerful influence and that it may trigger unexpected emotional reactions. This can happen particularly in individuals who no longer have the cognitive abilities to communicate verbally, and these emotional reactions may range from pleasant to distressful. Facial expressions, gestures, and body postures give indications of pleasant or distressful experiences and music therapists can follow these cues to know whether to reciprocate the emotion or to give comfort through touch, gestures, vocal inflection and/or physical proximity. A music therapist may also provide an opportunity for iconic representation of these emotions through drum beating, gestured movements, or vocal sounds, among other approaches. While all individuals can use iconic emotional representations in these ways, persons who are nonverbal due to inexperience or cognitive impairments have a particular need to use these nonverbal approaches. When facilitated by a qualified music therapist, these experiences provide emotional release and successful, socially appropriate, emotional expressions for those who do not have the capacities to express them in any other way.

Reality Orientation and Validation. Reality orientation, conceptualized by J. C. Folsom (Folsom, 1983), is considered by many as central to psychological well-being for persons who are elderly in many settings, particularly if they have memory lapses. Music therapists often incorporate reality orientation in some form into many of their sessions, but caution must be exercised concerning whether or not it is an appropriate approach to use with all persons who are elderly. With an emphasis on awareness of person, place and time, reality orientation is suitable for those persons who have sufficient cognitive ability to process the information. It is not suitable for those who do not have such ability. These include those who have severe losses of memory due to dementia, or other cognitive impairments. For them, each piece of information is new, as if they are hearing it for the first time. Sometimes the news, though reality, is devastating each time it is presented, e.g., for a woman with severe dementia who asked every day if her husband was coming to visit only to be told each time that he was dead. With each orientation to reality this woman's reaction of intense grief was repeated and its' contribution to her well-being was questionable when medication was required to calm her agitation.

In cases such as this, it may be most helpful to validate a belief (Feil, 1989). This may be controversial since validation of belief is not completely truthful, but such validation need not be false. Music therapists and other helping professionals may have told the lady with concern for her husband's visit that he was not coming today and that she had been left in their care while he was gone. Such a statement is true, yet it is not distressing.

Musical Skills and Aesthetic Experiences as Values in Aging. To enhance well-being, some people who are elderly use music skills, to structure time alone, stimulate their intellects, express emotions, engage in social contact with others, receive affirmations from their peers, and provide entertainment for themselves and for others. To reach these ends, adults in their late years often have the desire to redevelop musical skills from their pasts, or to develop entirely new ones. Though they have the interest, opportunities for entry level skill development are frequently nonexistent. These limitations are due to cultural biases which preclude learning new skills in advanced years, little knowledge concerning educational techniques and methods, and little or no commitment from traditional music educators to teach music throughout the life span. Yet, individuals who have had opportunities for music skill development in their 7th and 8th decades have found them very therapeutic (Gibbons, 1984).

Though persons who are elderly can have successes with musical skill development and maintenance, it is essential that any program designed for a specific person must have goals that are realistic for that person. While it may not be critical that such a program be offered by a music therapist, it is the music therapist who is most often open and willing to provide a music development opportunity for an older person. It is also the music therapist who will likely develop a nontraditional approach to meet program goals because it is the one that best suits that individual's desires, strengths, and needs.

As in all programs designed and implemented by music therapists, the individual consumer must have input into defining the desired outcomes and the processes by which they will be achieved. Music therapists also have a responsibility to exercise caution and to advise against musical participation that is contraindicated. Included in the contraindications are (1) wind instruments for persons who have hypertension since the resistance of blowing an instrument increases blood pressure, (2) instruments that require great finger dexterity in those who have physically limiting conditions such as arthritis, and, also for these persons, (3) instruments that require physical pressure to hold and/or to play such as a violin, viola, or cello, among others.

Whether a person who is elderly plays an instrument, sings, or otherwise participates in music, the value of music lies in aesthetic experience. Such value is demonstrated through the pervasiveness of music in all cultures of the world and throughout the daily lives of most people in those cultures. It is the aesthetic qualities of music that makes it unique, something quite out of the ordinary, and something which fulfills the need to experience the beautiful. These aesthetic qualities offer escape from the human condition, all the while they enhance being human. They can be experienced alone or with others, and music is flexible so that a skilled music therapist can adjust these qualities to suit those who have varying physical, psychological, social, and spiritual response levels.

Of course, the aesthetic experience is not the same for each individual and it is not experienced with the same music. The best facilitator of the aesthetic experience is the music that is preferred by the individual person in a particular setting, for a particular purpose, and at a particular time. Sometimes it is this aesthetic experience alone, without the structure of the music therapist's programming, that is pleasurable; but, it is the music therapist who can direct an individual's focus, perception, cognition, and affect to achieve specific or extended therapeutic value (Gfeller, 1990).

Spiritual Values in Aging

Many persons in their later years are very interested in confirming their spiritual beliefs or in enhancing their spiritual lives in some way. That is not to say, however, that all persons who are elderly have such spiritual interests, and it must not be assumed that all persons should have to deal with spiritual matters in their later years. Again, the role of a facilitator in spirituality, including the music therapist, must be determined by the person who is requesting the intervention. This role may involve a range of functions from providing familiar music to designing musical experiences which are intended to enhance meditation or prayer. In determining these functions, individuals may be more or less articulate concerning their desires, but the music therapist must seek their input for preferred outcomes and the strategies to reach them. Sometimes this is expressed as a desire to manage anxiety and fear of the unknown, or it is the desire to develop or deepen a relationship with a deity; however that is defined by an individual.

Though spirituality is not the same as religious practice or beliefs, the belief system of the individual is central to spiritual program design. It is therefore essential that the music therapist understand well the belief systems of individuals with whom they work and their cultural contexts. It is also essential that the music therapist realize that not all persons who subscribe to a particular belief system will actualize it in the same ways, i.e., some may immerse themselves in religious rituals while others may find rituals disdainful.

For those music therapists who are open and interested in spiritual development with older individuals but who do not feel confident as a spiritual director, it is possible to work in conjunction with a chaplain or another qualified person who can assume primary responsibility for guiding spiritual growth. Here the music therapist can make appropriate music selections to facilitate experiences in a wide range of spiritual contexts. The music therapist can also provide information and training concerning the use of music in these contexts.

INFORMED CONSENT

Central to all codes of ethics, including the one for music therapists, is informed consent (Corey, Corey, & Callanan, 1988). Probably, the best assurance that client's rights are protected occurs when music therapists provide clear information about the nature of the therapy, its expected beneficial outcomes, and its possible deleterious effects. Included with this communication must be the rights and responsibilities of both the clients and the therapists. This information must be presented in language that is understood by the client, or the client's guardian. With this information, clients, or their guardians, can act freely to make rational decisions.

Guardians are requested to give informed consent for those who have relinquished legally their authority to give their own consent. This shift in authority may create problems if the individual does not want to participate in a research and/or clinical music therapy program, but cannot communicate this desire. The guardian or next of kin may consider the music therapy program beneficial, but the individual client may not have a positive response to it. The music therapist has the responsibility to observe carefully all participation, nonparticipation, and nonverbal communication in the client during procedures to determine if they are appropriate and if the client is receptive to them. If the client seems agitated, has a closed body posture with downcast eyes, and facial expressions that indicate disinterest, or even distress, the music therapist must terminate the procedure.

Music Therapy Intervention

Involvement and commitment to music therapy interventions must be based on informed consent given by the individual client or by the client's guardian. Prior to involvement in a music therapy intervention, the music therapist assesses an individual's strengths and needs and then develops an intervention which is designed to maintain and/or develop strengths while it meets the needs. Once the intervention is designed, it is communicated carefully to each individual. Subsequently, that individual must decide whether or not the intervention is desirable and whether or not a commitment will be made to participate in it. Individuals must make these decisions in consideration of as much information as possible concerning expected outcomes and any possible deleterious effects. Even if persons are debilitated to the point at which they are not verbal and it is questionable whether or not they understand, the music therapist must explain clearly and succinctly about the music therapy procedure, it's intended outcome, and how it will be conducted. In this circumstance, the individual's behaviors are observed to determine whether or not the program is appropriate, e.g., open or closed body posture, downcast or uplifted head, whether or not there is eye contact, facial expressions of pleasure or displeasure, and any indication of participation at the individual's physical, psychological, and social response levels.

In addition to projected therapeutic outcomes, individuals, or their caregivers, must also base the decision for music therapy participation on expected program duration and expected program costs. The duration is determined by the music therapist who sets a time line on service delivery. To do this the music therapist estimates as closely as possible the amount of time required for desired outcomes to occur. While this depends on individual responses, periodic evaluations of program effectiveness will provide information which contributes to the decision to continue or discontinue the program. If desired outcomes are not reached within a reasonable amount of time, the intervention must be discontinued. If, on the other hand, desirable outcomes are achieved, and continuation in music therapy is requested, another time defined period for service delivery can begin. This service, and any subsequent service delivery, depends on the assessment and evaluation of consistent and beneficial outcomes for the client, and a commitment from the music therapist to continue. If the music therapist determines at any point the therapeutic intervention is not viable and efficacious to the client, or that the relationship with the client is no longer desirable, there is a responsibility to end the intervention.

Program cost can influence the decision to begin or to continue with a music therapy intervention. The cost in terms of fees for services and the payment arrangements for the services, however they are determined, must be communicated clearly and agreed upon before music therapy services are initiated. Services must be time limited and changes in fee structure must not be imposed once they are initiated. At the conclusion of the time defined, service period, fees may be revised for subsequent periods.

Other program costs must also be communicated clearly before a commitment is made. These include the amount of time each session will take, the number of sessions per week, what responsibilities the individual clients must assume, and considerations for travel to and from the sessions.

Once the decision is made for music therapy program involvement, the professional music therapist must consider individual clients' preferences for music and the ways in which it is used as integral to each person's program design. In addition, individuals must have as much control as possible over their levels of involvement, their responses to the music, and their freedom to choose whether they will or will not continue in the program.

Music Therapy Research

A qualified music therapist works to design interventions from a basis of theory and knowledge derived from research and efficacious practice models. This knowledge guides practice and it is from practice that research grows to further expand and disseminate knowledge in the field. Without theory and knowledge from research, practice is random, or it relies on intuition.

While research is integral to effective practice, it must comply with the Code of Ethics (National Association for Music Therapy, 1987) and it must be conducted only with those persons who have given their informed consent. These individuals, therefore, have a full understanding of the procedures that will be used, the possible benefits, and any associated risks. There must be no deception in the administration of research programs.

The individuals who give consent to participate in research must be competent to make the decision to participate, must volunteer with the understanding that they may withdraw their participation at any time, and must fully comprehend what they are about to do (National Association for Music Therapy Code of Ethics, 1987). In addition, the participant's identity must be protected and confidentiality maintained. In the case of relinquished authority to give consent, the guardian must give informed consent after indicating a clear understanding of procedures, and anticipated outcomes.

Video and Audio Recordings

Informed consent must be obtained to use any video or audio tape recordings of clients in music therapy sessions. Whether these recordings are intended for use in research data collection, academic or public education, or for any other use, each individual involved must fully understand the purpose and must give consent by signature to use the recordings for that explicit purpose. Again, guardians may give informed consent for those who cannot give their own. In no circumstances may the music therapist use the recordings in any way other than that specified on the signed, informed consent form.

CONCLUSION

The field of music therapy has a Code of Ethics and Standards for Clinical Practice which provide guidelines for making ethical decisions including those that concern whether or not to engage, continue, or change treatment interventions with particular clients, among others. Those guidelines, however, are general in scope and do not provide all answers to ethical questions concerning client treatment. Music therapists, then, have a responsibility to know themselves, to be aware of their strengths and abilities, to know their boundaries and to be secure in their values. In the framework of this self knowledge, the individual music therapist must make decisions which are ethical. As music therapists practice with full awareness of their values, knowledge, skills, and abilities, it is essential to document all clients' processes through therapeutic interventions, and to seek counsel from other experienced professionals when issues of ethical concern are raised. While this approach does not guarantee ethical decisions in music therapy practice, it assures them to the greatest degree possible.

REFERENCES

Clair, A. & Bernstein, B. (1990a). A comparison of singing, vibrotactile and nonvibrotactile instrumental playing responses in severely regressed persons with dementia of the Alzheimer's type. *Journal of Music Therapy, 27*, 119-125.

Clair, A. & Bernstein, B. (1990b). A preliminary study of music therapy programming for severely regressed persons with Alzheimer's type dementia. *Journal of Applied Gerontology, 9*, 299-311.

Corey, G., Corey, M., & Callanan, P. (1988). *Issues and ethics in the helping professions*. (3rd. ed.) Pacific Grove, CA: Brooks/Cole Publishing Company.

Feil, N. (1989). *Validation*. (Revised ed.) Cleveland, OH: Edward Feil Productions.

Folsom, J. C. (1983). Reality orientation. In B. Reisberg (Ed.), *Alzheimer's disease: The standard reference*. (pp. 449-454). New York: The Free Press.

Gaston, E. T. (1968). Music is human behavior. In E. T. Gaston (Ed.), *Music in Therapy*. (pp. 7-29). New York: Macmillan Publishing Company.

Gfeller, K. E. (1990). The function of aesthetic stimuli in the therapeutic process. In R. F. Unkefer (Ed.), *Music therapy in the treatment of adults with mental disorders*. (pp. 70- 81). New York: Schirmer Books.

Gibbons, A. C. (1984). A music therapy program for non-institutionalized, mature adults: A description. *Activities, Adaptation and Aging, 6*, 71-80.

Jonsen, A. R., Siegler, M. & Winslade, W. J. (1982). *Clinical ethics a practical approach to ethical decisions in clinical medicine*. New York: Macmillan Publishing Company, Inc.

McIntosh, G., Thaut, M., Rice, R., & Prassas, S. (1993). Auditory rhythmic cueing in gait rehabilitation with stroke patients. *Canadian Journal of Neurological Sciences, 20* (Suppl. 4), 168.

Moranto, C., Wheeler, B. (1986). Teaching ethics in music therapy. *Music Therapy Perspectives, 3*, 17-19.

National Association for Music Therapy Code of Ethics (1987). The National Association for Music Therapy, Silver Spring, MD.

National Association for Music Therapy Standards of Clinical Practice (1987). The National Association for Music Therapy, Silver Spring, MD.

Thaut, M., Schleiffers, S. & Davis, W. (1992) Changes in EMG patterns under the influence of auditory rhythm. In R. Spintge & R. Droh (Eds.), *Music Medicine.* (pp.80-101). St. Louis: MMB Music, Inc.

Wylie, M. E. (1990). A comparison of the effects of old familiar songs, antique objects, historical summaries, and general questions on the reminiscence of nursing home residents. *Journal of Music Therapy, 27,* 2-12.

CAREGIVING

Ethical Challenges Facing Family Caregivers of Persons with Alzheimer's Disease

Karen A. Roberto

SUMMARY. Alzheimer's disease is a progressive, irreversible neurological disorder that robs individuals of their cognitive and functional capabilities. The basic principles of bioethics, beneficence, autonomy and paternalism, and justice, provide the framework for understanding the issues and situations that challenge family caregivers as they make decisions that influence the well-being of their loved ones. Practitioners can play an active role in helping caregivers effectively negotiate within and between these ethical constructs as they provide care for their family members.

Alzheimer's disease is a progressive, irreversible neurological disorder that robs individuals of their cognitive and functional capabilities. It affects more than two million Americans with its incidence increasing from less than one percent for individuals under age 65 to more than ten percent for persons 65 years of age and older (Evans et al., 1989). As people are living longer, the prevalence of Alzheimer's disease is likely to increase.

Cognitive impairment is the hallmark of Alzheimer's disease. As a person moves through the stages of the disease, his or her memory, problem solving skills, judgement, comprehension, atten-

Karen A. Roberto, PhD, is Professor and Coordinator, Gerontology Program, University of Northern Colorado, Greeley, CO 80639.

[Haworth co-indexing entry note]: "Ethical Challenges Facing Family Caregivers of Persons with Alzheimer's Disease." Roberto, Karen A. Co-published simultaneously in *Activities, Adaptation & Aging* (The Haworth Press, Inc.) Vol. 18, No. 3/4, 1994, pp. 49-61; and: *Ethics and Values in Long Term Health Care* (ed: Patricia J. Villani) The Haworth Press, Inc., 1994, pp. 49-61. Multiple copies of this article/chapter may be purchased from The Haworth Document Delivery Center [1-800-3-HAWORTH; 9:00 a.m. - 5:00 p.m. (EST)].

49

tion-span, and language abilities diminish. These intellectual deficits, in addition to any coexisting physical and emotional conditions, limits the person's ability to perform routine activities of daily living. In the early to mid-stages of the disease, the person has difficulty accomplishing instrumental tasks such as shopping, cleaning, cooking, and handling money. In the latter stages, as cognitive abilities further decline, the person requires assistance with more personal tasks such as bathing, dressing, and toileting.

Family members are the primary source of care and support for older individuals with long-term, disabling health conditions such as Alzheimer's disease. The primary caregiver tends to be a spouse, who assumes the role of caregiver at a time in their life when they may be experiencing their own health problems or the reduction of functional capacities associated with aging (Cantor, 1983; Johnson, 1983). When a spouse is not available or is unable to provide care, adult children, most frequently daughters or daughters-in-law, assume the caregiving responsibilities for their aging parents (Stone, Cafferate, & Sangl, 1987).

During the course of their caregiving career, family members encounter various situations that require them to make ethical and value-ridden decisions related to the care and well-being of their loved ones. The personal value system of the caregiver serves as the ultimate basis for the care provided to the individual with Alzheimer's disease (McGovern, 1991). Specifically, caregivers' beliefs about (a) their family member, (b) the disease, and (c) death and dying influence their decision-making processes and the types of interventions or treatments they institute.

Many of the issues and dilemmas facing caregivers place them in the center of a double-bind situation; the decision to act or not act is emotionally painful and guilt-provoking. The basic principles of bioethics, beneficence, autonomy and paternalism, and justice, provide the framework from which to examine the issues and situations that challenge family caregivers of persons with Alzheimer's disease.

BENEFICENCE

One of the primary moral imperatives of our society is that we be beneficent; that is charitable and kind. Applied to family caregiving situations, beneficence can be viewed as the caregiver's role in promoting good and preventing harm and suffering in the life of the care receiver (Hasselkus, 1991; Turnbull, 1990). These two aspects of this principle often come into conflict with one another. For example, wandering, a common behavior of persons with Alzheimer's disease, creates a situation where caregivers often feel uneasy about or fear for the safety of their family members. One means of controlling this behavior is by the use of either physical or chemical restraints. For some individuals, restraints have a calming effect while for others they may increase their level of restlessness or induce agitation (Mace & Rabins, 1991). Whether or not to use a restraint is a difficult decision for most caregivers as they strive to find a balance between maintaining the dignity and independence and safety and security of their care receivers.

Fear of violating the principles of beneficence is a predominant concern among caregivers. In an ethnographic study of 15 caregivers of older adults, nursing home placement was viewed as the most clearcut and powerful representation of violation (Hasselkus & Stetson, 1991). The caregivers believed that nursing home placement would result in inferior care and that institutionalization would inevitably precipitate further physical and psychological deterioration in their care receivers. Yet, typically in the mid- to final stages of Alzheimer's disease, caregivers recognize that nursing home placement is beneficial and "for the good" of their loved ones. The decision to institutionalize is not made hastily, however, and often is a product of years of consideration as guilt over past conversations and promises never to subject the elder to life in a nursing home often reinforces the caregiver's reluctance to seriously consider this care option (Colerick & George, 1986; Pruchino, Michaels, & Potashnik, 1990).

In the final stages of Alzheimer's disease, persons are often confined to bed, incontinent, and unable to express themselves (Mace & Rabins, 1991). Family members responsible for their care and well-being frequently wrestle with issues surrounding the "quality of life" of their loved ones while struggling with their own feelings of stress, burden, and despair. Moody (1992) views caregivers in this situation as facing one of the temptations of beneficence–beneficent euthanasia. He suggests that "the danger of beneficence is that there are powerful attractions to killing people, particularly to overburdened caregivers who begin to think of the patient as already dead" (p. 47). Although criminal law prohibits deliberately taking the life of another, even if motivated by compassion, passive euthanasia is more generally accepted (Turnbull, 1990). Amidst their grieving for the loss of the person they once knew, caregivers must make difficult decisions as to what and how much life support should be given; an often complex and troubling dilemma associated with Alzheimer's disease.

AUTONOMY AND PATERNALISM

Autonomy

Central to the issue of autonomy is the older person's competence and freedom to make choices and execute decisions in a manner consistent with his or her values (Cicirelli, 1992). To be autonomous suggests that the person is capable of rational thought. When cognitive abilities are impaired, caregivers often must make and execute decisions for the welfare of their family members. To avoid conflict between caregiver respect for autonomy and caregiver paternalism, the level of the elder's decisional and executional capacity must be carefully assessed (Cicirelli, 1992). This is an especially difficult task for caregivers of family members in the early- to mid-stages of Alzheimer's disease whose decision-making capacity fluctuates across time and situations.

Since it is possible for individuals to be capable of autonomous decision-making in some areas of their lives and not others, the meaning of autonomy for older adults with Alzheimer's disease needs to be broadened to consider several sub-types or levels of autonomy rather than focusing on one particular aspect or interpretation. For example, Collopy (1988, p. 11) identified six polarities within autonomy: (a) *decisional–executive*: having preferences, making decisions versus being able to implement them or carry them out; (b) *direct–delegated*: deciding or acting on one's own versus giving authority to others to decide or act; (c) *competent–incapacitated*: reasonably and judgmentally coherent choice or activity versus that which exhibits rational defect or judgmental incoherence; (d) *authentic–inauthentic*: choices or actions which are consonant with character versus those which are seriously out of character; (e) *immediate–long range*: present or limited expressions of autonomy versus future or wide-ranging expressions; and (f) *negative–positive*: choice or activity that claims a right only to non-interference versus that which claims positive entitlement, support, or capacitation. Similarly, Cicirelli (1992) proposed examining autonomy on a continuum from *direct autonomy,* where the person depends on his or her existing information and capacity to make and execute decisions, to *surrogate autonomy* which occurs when the individual is no longer capable of making decisions on his or her own, but the caregiver attempts to make the decision in the way that the care receiver would if he or she were able.

As suggested by both these perspectives, autonomous decision-making for persons with declining cognitive abilities need not be denied, but rather enhanced through their participation in the decision-making process. As the individual's mental and physical abilities decline, the caregiver will need to take a more active role in the decision-making process. An examination of decisional autonomy and decision-making processes among elderly single mothers and their caregiving daughters found that increased levels of dependency for personal care led to the decreased confidence in their decision-making abilities and higher levels of daughters' influence over decisions (Pratt, Jones, Shin, & Walker, 1989). Daughters reported that declines in the mothers' health status was a major reason for their increased role in decision making.

A common concern of caregivers of family members with Alzheimer's disease is the preservation of autonomy when the care receivers become too mentally incapacitated to make decisions for themselves. Their rights to self-determination can best be upheld by involving them in the decision-making process that addresses their future welfare (McGovern, 1991). Ideally, long-term care decisions are made prior to the onset of Alzheimer's disease or at least during the early stages of the disease when the person has the greatest level of cognitive competency. This requires, however, that the person be told his or her diagnosis. This issue faces most family caregivers, particularly in the early stages of the disease. Dubler (1987) argues that persons not told about their condition are disempowered and "that without that knowledge, there is no way to ferret out, to document, and to give respect to the individual's personal preferences for care" (p. 13).

Disagreements arise, however, concerning how much autonomy should be granted the prior wishes of the person. Dyck (1984) points out that in a slowly progressing disease, such as Alzheimer's disease, there are various points at which judgement will need to be made as to whether the next life-sustaining procedure is one the person would have preferred to avoid. He argues for "consensus management" whereby all caregivers concerned with the care of the person (i.e., family members, medical personnel) be in consensus to serve the best interests of the impaired individual.

Conversely, Veatch (1984) suggests that for individuals who were formerly competent and who have expressed their wishes for terminal care, family caregivers should use "substituted judgement" to carry-out the loved one's wishes. In this type of situation, the caregiver "takes into account idiosyncratic factors that the person has expressed with the goal of honoring his or her wishes" (p. 667). If the person's wishes were never stated, Veatch argues that "the family must choose among the reasonable courses of action that are available, not necessarily the single definitive best course" (p. 668). He proposes a principle of "limited family autonomy" where the family is presumed guardian with the limited authority to choose the values of its incompetent members until it appears that the family is going too far beyond reason, in which case the courts must get involved. In support of this notion, Kapp (1987) suggests that "intervention should go no further than it absolutely must in order to accomplish its legitimate aims. Thus, means of substitute decision-making that least deprive the resident of respect for autonomy are favored over more extensive interventions" (p. 271).

Paternalism

A paternalistic act occurs when a caregiver decides to override the autonomous choice of the care receiver (Hogstel & Gaul, 1991). Some individuals argue that paternalism is never justified; others suggest that under certain circumstances it can be justified by reasons related to the welfare, good, happiness, or values of the person being coerced (Dworkin, 1972; Gert & Culver, 1979). Three co-existing conditions are necessary to justify paternalism: (a) the harm prevented or benefit provided to the person must outweigh the loss of independence; (b) the condition of the person must severely limit the ability of autonomous choice; and (c) the action must be universally justified (Beauchamp & Childress, 1983).

Moody (1992) contends that when caring for a person with Alzheimer's disease, actions favoring paternalism may sometimes be pragmatic in situations where its purpose is to maintain the person's self-respect. For example, to avoid unnecessary humiliation, a caregiver may pre-arrange to have groceries charged to his or her personal account and allow the person with Alzheimer's disease to continue in the "shopper" role by paying for groceries with fake or "monopoly" money. Another common, face-saving technique used by caregivers is to request that the physician order the impaired person to stop driving rather than the caregiver taking the keys away (Mace & Rabins, 1991; Moody, 1992). In both these situations, paternalistic intervention is accompanied by deception to preserve the dignity of the person with Alzheimer's disease.

JUSTICE

Justice is the search for the "ethically appropriate way to spread limited resources though the moral community" (Veatch, 1981, p. 254). At a more micro level, justice in caregiving involves two separate, but related issues: (a) balancing the needs of the care receiver with those of the caregiver, and (b) sharing the responsibility for care among family members.

Commonly adhered to by family caregivers are the principles suggested by Rawls's *Maximum Theory of Justice*. This theory purports that persons seek to maximize the net benefits of members of society who are the most burdened and the least advantaged (Veatch, 1981). When caring for family members with Alzheimer's disease, caregivers often suppress their own needs in order to meet those of their care receivers. Caregiving restricts their use of personal time (Kleban, Brody, Shoonover, & Hoffman, 1989; Montgomery, Gonyea, & Hooyman, 1985), interferes with employment responsibilities and obligations (Stone et al., 1987; Young & Kahana, 1989) and strains family relationships (Scott, Roberto, Hutton, & Slack, 1985; Stephens, Kinney, & Ogrocki, 1991). As a result, caregivers report emotional distress, burden, and stress as they strive to fulfill their familial responsibilities (Gallagher, Wrabetz, Lovett, Maestro, & Rose 1988; Quayhagen & Quayhagen, 1988; Zarit, Orr, & Zarit, 1985).

The second issue of justice in caregiving, the sharing of the responsibility for care among family members, emerges when caregivers feel a sense of unfair responsibility and lack of support from others (Hasselkus & Stetson, 1991). The structure of most caregiving networks is hierarchical with one member of the immediate family assuming the role of primary care provider. Questions of spousal and filial responsibilities arise, especially when there are several siblings involved (Mace & Rabins, 1991), as families struggle with the problems of equity or fairness in the distribution of caregiving burden. Moody (1992) asserts that the "resolution of questions about distributive justice will depend on whether the family can achieve a measure of free and open communications about the problem they are facing" (p. 61).

IMPLICATIONS FOR PRACTITIONERS

The nature of the issues involved in providing care for a family member with Alzheimer's disease invoke strong emotions and challenge the moral assumptions of all concerned. Practitioners working with family caregivers must recognize and understand the ethical dilemmas facing these individuals and assist them in clarifying their personal values and beliefs.

One of the first issues facing caregivers is whether or not to tell family members the diagnosis. Under the principle of autonomy, the person is seen as having a moral right to know; adherence to the principles of beneficence may lead to the decision to withhold this information if it is felt that it would be detrimental to the well-being of the individual (Turnbull, 1990). When asked, the majority of individuals indicate they would want to be informed of the diagnosis as it would allow them to plan for financial and personal care, seek a second opinion, and settle family matters (Erde, Nadal, & Scholl, 1988). Health and human service professionals need to be sensitive to caregivers' concerns about disclosing the truth and help them assess the benefits as well of costs of informing their family members of their diagnosis.

Caregivers often have difficulty deciding what is best for the well-being of their care receivers in light of the possible dangers they may confront. For example, in the early- to mid-stages of the disease process, the caregiver may struggle with questions such as: (a) Can the person manage his or her own money? (b) Should he or she continue to do the cooking? (c) Is it safe for him or her to drive? and (d) Should the person be left home alone? Practitioners can assist caregivers in objectively assessing each situation so that decisions to promote or restrict activities are made based on accurate and complete information. Time spent educating caregivers about potential effective strategies for helping their family members maintain as much independence as possible, without compromising their safety, can help alleviate their fears of doing "no harm" and enhance their abilities to "do good" for all involved (Hasselkus, 1991).

To help guide families through their caregiving careers, professionals should encourage long-term planning in relationship to service options and living arrangements for their loved ones. Caregivers often lack the information they need to make informed choices for the care of their family members. Social service providers have the knowledge to assist them in accessing services appropriate for their relatives and themselves. In addition, they usually have professional contacts that are a source of information about the *quality* of facilities or services that generally is not available to family caregivers (U.S. Congress, Office of Technology Assessment, 1990). This information needs to be shared with caregivers so that they can accurately evaluate different care options.

As the disease progresses, and the individual's cognitive abilities deteriorate, caregivers play a more active role in making health care decisions on behalf of their family members. This role often collides with the principles of autonomy that imply that individuals have the right to decide on the type and level of care that they want implemented (Cassel & Goldstein, 1988). Caregivers can help uphold their care receivers rights by helping them establish and make known their choices and preferences while they are still able to choose. Practitioners need to encourage caregivers to document advance directive strategies (e.g., living wills, health care proxy) as a means of ensuring that these choices are respected by medical personnel (Cassel & Goldstein, 1988) as well as by other family members (Malloy, Clarnette, Braun, Eisemann, & Sneiderman, 1991).

Caring for a person with Alzheimer's disease over a long period of time induces stress and strain in the lives of most family caregivers. Professionals need to frequently remind caregivers to take care of themselves, especially in the mid- to later stages of the disease, when they typically become more caught up in providing for the needs of their care receivers than for their own health and emotional well-being (Ballard, 1989). Encouraging caregivers to allow family members to attend adult day care programs, for example, provides them respite from the constant care and oversight of their loved ones. Participating in a support group also can be beneficial for caregivers as they often learn new strategies for coping with changes in their care receivers' abilities and behaviors as well as providing them with an opportunity to express their feelings among others facing similar circumstances.

Long-established roles, responsibilities, and expectations within the family influences who takes on the primary responsibility of caring for the older person with Alzheimer's disease. Practitioners should encourage family members to share responsibility for care so that a single individual is not forced to bear the entire burden of care (Wetle et al., 1989). Although one person may be designated to provide daily care, other family members can assist by taking over some of the tasks that use to be performed by the person with Alzheimer's disease, gathering information about care options, and providing short-term respite for the primary caregiver.

In conclusion, caregivers need the support of both health and human service professionals as they confront the challenges and dilemmas of providing care for their family members with Alzheimer's disease. Practitioners will need to play multiple roles (e.g., information provider, counselor, advocate) as they help caregivers through the process of negotiation within and between ethical principles in an effort to help maintain beneficence, autonomy, and justice for their care receivers and themselves (Hasselkus & Stetson, 1991).

REFERENCES

Ballard, E. (1989). Support systems: Meeting the needs of patients and family caregivers coping with Alzheimer's disease. *Physical Therapy in Health Care, 2*(3/4), 41-52.

Beauchamp, T., & Childress, J. (1983). *Principles of biomedical ethics.* New York: Oxford University Press.

Cantor, M. (1983). Strain among caregivers: A study of experience in the United States. *The Gerontologist, 23,* 597-604.

Cassel, C., & Goldstein, K. (1988). Ethical considerations. In L. Jarvik & C. Winograd (Eds.), *Treatments for the Alzheimer's patient* (pp. 80-104). New York: Springer.

Cicirelli, V. (1992). *Family caregiving: Autonomous and paternalistic decision making.* Newbury Park, CA: Sage.

Colerick, E., & George, L. (1986). Predictors of institutionalization among caregivers of patients with Alzheimer's disease. *Journal of the American Geriatrics Society, 34,* 493-498.

Collopy, B. (1988). Autonomy in long-term care: Some crucial distinctions. *The Gerontologist, 28*(Supplement), 10-17.

Dubler, N. (1987). The legal and ethical dilemma. In A. Kalicki (Ed.), *Confronting Alzheimer's disease* (pp. 11-20). Owings Mills, MD: National Health Publishing.

Dworkin, G. (1972). Paternalism. *The Monist, 56,* 64-84.

Dyck, A. (1984). Ethical aspects of care for the dying incompetent. *Journal of the American Geriatrics Society, 32,* 661-664.

Erde, E., Nadal, E., & Scholl, T. (1988). On truth telling and the diagnosis of Alzheimer's disease. *Journal of Family Practice, 28,* 401-406.

Evans, D., Funkenstein, H., Albert, M., Scherr, P., Cook, N., Chown, M., Herbert, L., Hennekens, C., & Taylor, J. (1989). Prevalence of Alzheimer's disease in a community population of older persons. *Journal of the American Medical Association, 262,* 2551-2556.

Gallagher, D., Wrabetz, A., Lovett, S., Maestro, S., & Rose, J. (1988). Depression and other negative affects in family caregivers. In E. Light & B. Lebowitz (Eds.), *Alzheimer's disease treatment and family stress: Directions for research* (pp. 218-244). Washington, DC: U.S. Government Printing Office.

Gert, B., & Culver, C. (1979). The justification of paternalism. In W. Robison & M. Pritchard (Eds.), *Medical responsibility* (pp. 1-4). Clifton, NJ: Humana Press.

Hasselkus, B. (1991). Ethical dilemmas in family caregiving for the elderly: Implications for occupational therapy. *American Journal of Occupational Therapy, 45,* 206-212.

Hasselkus, B., & Stetson, S. (1991). Ethical dilemmas: The organization of family caregiving for the elderly. *Journal of Aging Studies, 5*(1), 99-110.

Hogstel, M., & Gaul, A. (1991). Safety or autonomy: An ethical issue for clinical gerontological nurses. *Journal of Gerontological Nursing, 17*(3), 6-11.

Johnson, C. (1983). Dyadic family relations and social support. *The Gerontologist, 23,* 610-618.

Kapp, M. (1987). Family decision-making for nursing home residents: Legal mechanisms and ethical underpinnings. *Theoretical Medicine, 8,* 259-273.

Kleban, M., Brody, E., Shoonover, C., & Hoffman, C. (1989). Family help to the elderly: Perceptions of sons-in-law regarding parent care. *Journal of Marriage and the Family, 51,* 303-312.

Mace, N., & Rabins, P. (1991). *The 36-hour day (revised ed.).* Baltimore, MD: The Johns Hopkins University Press.

Malloy, D., Clarnette, R., Braun, E., Eisemann, M., & Sneiderman, B. (1991). Decision making in the incompetent elderly: "The daughter from California syndrome." *Journal of the American Geriatrics Society, 39,* 396-399.

McGovern, T. (1991). Ethical considerations. In R. L. Dippel & J. T. Hutton (Eds.), *Caring for the Alzheimer patient (2nd ed.)* (pp. 169-177). Buffalo, NY: Golden Age Books.

Montgomery, R., Gonyea, J., & Hooyman, N. (1985). Caregiving and the experience of subjective and objective burden. *Family Relations, 34,* 19-26.

Moody, H.R. (1992). *Ethics in an aging society.* Baltimore, MD: The Johns Hopkins University Press.

Pratt, C., Jones, L., Shin, H., & Walker, A. (1989). Autonomy and decision making between single older women and their caregiving daughters. *The Gerontologist, 29,* 792-797.

Pruchino, R., Michaels, E., & Potashnik, S. (1990). Predictors of institutionalization among Alzheimer's disease victims with caregiving spouses. *Journal of Gerontology: Social Sciences, 45,* 259-266.

Quayhagen, M., & Quayhagen, M. (1988). Alzheimer's stress: Coping with the caregiving role. *The Gerontologist, 28,* 391-396.

Scott, J., Roberto, K., Hutton, J. T., Slack, D. (1985). Family conflicts in caring for the Alzheimer's patient. In J. T. Hutton & A.D. Kenny (Eds.), *Senile dementia of the Alzheimer type* (pp. 77-86). New York: Alan R. Liss.

Stephens, M., Kinney, J., Ogrocki, P. (1991). Stress and well-being among caregivers to older adults with dementia: The in-home versus nursing home experience. *The Gerontologist, 31,* 217-223.

Stone, R., Cafferate, G., & Sangl, J. (1987). Caregivers of the frail elderly: A national profile. *The Gerontologist, 27,* 616-626.

Turnbull, S. (1990). Ethical issues in the care of the patient with Alzheimer's disease. In R. Hamdy, J. Turnbull, L. Norman., & M. Lancaster (Eds.), *Alzheimer's disease: A handbook for caregivers* (pp. 85-93). St. Louis: C. V. Mosby.

U.S. Congress, Office of Technology Assessment (1990). *Confused minds, burdened families: Finding help for people with Alzheimer's & other dementias.* Washington, DC: Government Printing Office.

Veatch, R. (1981). *A theory of medical ethics.* New York: Basic Books.

Veatch, R. (1984). An ethical framework for terminal care decisions: A new classification of patients. *Journal of the American Geriatrics Society, 32,* 665- 669.

Wetle, T., Besdine, R., Keckch, W., Morgan, H., Gesino, J., Smolski, S., & Fulmer, T. (1989). Family-centered detection and management of Alzheimer's disease. *Pride Institute of Long Term Health Care, 8*(4), 3-11.

Young, R. & Kahana, E. (1989). Specifying caregiver outcomes: Gender and relationship aspects of caregiving strain. *The Gerontologist, 29,* 660-666.

Zarit, S., Orr, N., & Zarit, J. (1985). *The hidden victims of Alzheimer's disease: Families under stress.* New York: New York University Press.

END OF LIFE CHOICES

Final Life Choices:
Who Decides?

Rosalie D. Marinelli

The trouble with mankind is that no one will admit that the main fact of existence is death . . . because man has a thinking brain and the longest lifetime, they are capable of the most horrible, long-term suffering . . . Is it humane to allow intense suffering to continue?

−72 year old woman, 1989

I will neither give a deadly drug to anyone if asked for it, nor will I make a suggestion to this effect

−Hippocratic oath

Rosalie D. Marinelli, EdD, is Associate Professor, Department of Health Sciences, University of Reno, NV. Her experience as a health educator in various health care settings has fostered an intense interest in ethical dilemmas.

The author wishes to express her appreciation to those who contributed to this article by agreeing to read the journal and be interviewed: Gleda Baldini, MD, Family Physician, Board certified in geriatrics, Manorville, NY; Annette Ballentine, Caregiver, Reno, NV; Peggy Bruhn, CSW, Bereavement Therapist, Port Jefferson, NY; Robert B. Burn, Jr., President and Chief Executive Officer, Washoe Health System, Reno, NV; Ann Griffith, LCSW, Clinical Social Worker, V.A. Medical Center, Reno, NV; Timothy E. Quill, MD, Internist, Rochester, NY; Barbara C. Thornton, PhD, Bioethicist, University of Nevada, Reno.

[Haworth co-indexing entry note]: "Final Life Choices: Who Decides?" Marinelli, Rosalie D. Co-published simultaneously in *Activities, Adaptation & Aging* (The Haworth Press, Inc.) Vol. 18, No. 3/4, 1994, pp. 65-76; and: *Ethics and Values in Long Term Health Care* (ed: Patricia J. Villani) The Haworth Press, Inc., 1994, pp. 65-76. Multiple copies of this article/chapter may be purchased from The Haworth Document Delivery Center [1-800-3-HAWORTH; 9:00 a.m. - 5:00 p.m. (EST)].

BACKGROUND

The first quote above is from the journal of a woman who died two and a half months after writing these words. Her journal was given to several persons from different disciplines and experiences who were asked to react to it–the chief executive officer of a hospital, a medical social worker in a Veterans Administration Hospital, an internist who has written extensively on death with dignity, a family practitioner in a skilled nursing facility, a bioethicist, a bereavement therapist, and a caregiver. In my role as interviewer, we discussed final life choices, who makes the decisions, and the ethical dimensions of dying, using the journal content as a stimulus. The opinions offered during these separate interviews are presented here, along with those of the author.

The Journal

How can one think and react to life normally when all about one is chaos and why do people who can do something about it if they are humane do not? I used to believe I had the ability to express ideas but I now see it is so terribly difficult when one is trying to express what has not been often discussed.

It is the men who have made all the laws–one has only to view the cruelty that occurs and the terrible suffering. Women have not had much say. I think we have now reached a time when the subject of Euthanasia can be discussed . . . [I can see why] the Euthanasia society is made up mostly of women in their sixties.

Imagine this if you can–all about you are people doing things they believe are the "right things to do," and they are *wrong*! Doing what is wrong for another for the *right* reasons can never be *right* . . . for women are words–man is action and doing the things that are done only because men say they *should* or *can* [be done].

The Dialogue

In her journal this woman is speaking to: "All of us, particularly decision-makers, to her family, of course, but to all of us" stated the bioethicist. While the hospital administrator and family physician also agreed she was speaking to society in general, she is speaking, "Symbolically to mankind" said the family physician. "Speaking to God . . . No one is listening to her here" said the bereavement therapist. The internist thought that her comments were, "not directed at anyone. . . . putting her thoughts together in a journal . . .." The medical social worker agreed these were personal thoughts, but she also wanted the medical staff to hear her. "I get the sense her medical caregivers had changed frequently and she gets close . . . and they leave [which] impacts on her ability to cope."

The answers to her questions about chaos and humaneness are very complex – "it is a societal, cultural issue" stated the hospital executive. The family physician was not sure what "it" was she wanted fixed, "Is the pain, suffering physical? mental?" Should health care providers do something? ". . . try to address it at each level, but some things are not fixable," remarked the internist, continuing: "first we must acknowledge the person is suffering; it is not humane to turn your back and pretend it is not there . . . even if you cannot alleviate or resolve it." "I think she thinks she is making a case for euthanasia," said the family physician, "but she does not make a very good case for it." The family physician believed that not being prepared to face life alone, as this woman seems to be, is not a clear case for suicide. The caregiver presumed her questions could only be answered by society. She does not necessarily "want answers" said the bereavement therapist, "She's screaming out in her journal because there was no one else . . . [we need to] respond by listening." "What I'm always impressed by is how humane men are to their dogs," noted the bioethicist, "they have no trouble giving it a kind and humane death, often with a lot of affection, but they won't do that for people." Why is it easier to be ethical and caring in matters concerning animals than it is for humans? "I think we need to learn to do for people what we have long done for our dogs," she concluded.

The bereavement therapist and the caregiver both commented that she is mourning her lost role. The internist stated that perhaps, being a woman, "she's more relationship orientated. "Actors are men, and they don't seem to feel her pain." He continued, "She was wife, mother, homemaker; caring for others, making the family work. Now no one is caring for her; she is feeling abandoned." Said the bioethicist, "Rules about death have been made by men, she's very correct . . . women would not design a system like this. In the past death was much more personal . . . and women were in charge of the rituals." "She's depressed! Why isn't anyone treating the depression?" asked the bereavement therapist. Both the family physician and the internist ask, "is this a depression that might be treated?" Was it unethical for the medical staff not to treat the depression? "Older persons do beautifully in therapy" said the bereavement therapist, "she would have benefitted." The family physician remarked that she makes a strong "case for increased psychiatric care because of her extreme depression. I *do not* have a responsibility to help her die." Euthanasia should only be explored "after every other avenue . . . address the pain, the depression, her spiritual needs" stated the internist. Only rarely does [the patient] actually mean 'I want you to help me die'. The patient may not have "examined their inner motives or been able to express their feelings – so they say 'I want to die,'" agreed the family physician. However, continued the internist, "there may be no alternatives. A relationship needs to be established to explore other avenues first; physician assisted dying would only be the *last* resort." The family physician asked: "If we can fix everything, would a perfect life lead to a perfect death?". . . "people want to control death, to achieve a perfect death." [This patient] may be making the right decision "but for all the wrong reasons."

Who decides? Ultimately the patient decides was the conclusion of all of the respondents except the hospital administrator. This individual believes that society too has a responsibility and must decide, "the patient, the family are too emotionally involved, too guilt-ridden; it's a terrible burden to place on anyone or any family member." "Perhaps with the help of their clergy" added the bereavement therapist. Certainly not hospitals . . . "I would not go to a hospital if I wanted to make my own decisions," said the caregiver. "[Death] has become impersonal and bureaucratic systems," said the bioethicist, "Hospitals are bureaucracies, where people die of bureaucracy. Hospices, on the other hand, which generally had a female influence, are kind and caring." If others are intensely connected with the patient, they should be involved, "but the patient ultimately decides," added the internist. The basis of ethical considerations in life ending decisions is that the patient initiates and the patient decides.

All those who read this journal agreed that they personally, and society in general, had some responsibility to this woman. But they disagreed somewhat about the extent of their obligations. Euthanasia, assisted suicide, individual rights, professional obligations, are often competing decisions with even more complex responses.

INTRODUCTION

Since 1976 with the Karen Ann Quinlan case (Annas, 1990), the legal ramifications of dying have been prominently discussed. All states and the District of Columbia have passed "living wills" legislation (Caralis et al., 1993), though advance directives is a much more descriptive term and includes durable power of attorney. But, despite reported public enthusiasm for advance directives, few patients actually complete one (Emanuel, 1993). As for decision-making for incompetent or unconscious patients, in all but two states, a surrogate is allowed to make treatment decisions on behalf of that person (which was the basis of the Quinlan case).

The exceptions to the surrogate ruling are New York and Missouri (Annas, 1990). Even with these far-reaching rulings, the legal decisions have not been consistent, have not helped the pain of families nor the ethical deliberations for health professionals who still struggle with these complex issues (Cassel and Meier, 1990; Singer and Siegler, 1990). For example, in New Jersey, family members can make treatment decisions for an unconscious or incompetent person but across the river in New York state, they cannot.

As the respondents to the journal of a dying woman indicated, there are philosophical, legal, social, emotional, economical and moral concerns. The scope of this discussion is focused on ethical considerations, which may include all of the above.

PROFESSIONALS' DILEMMA

The two quotes, one from a dying woman and one from the "father of medicine," Hippocrates, seem to be on a course of direct conflict: the patient's wishes versus the physician's oath to give no deadly drugs. However, it must be noted that the woman was writing this journal in 1989, while the Hippocratic Oath is over 2500 years old. Many medical schools no longer administer this oath when granting a medical degree.

The case for physicians' intervention in the process of dying by either active euthanasia or assisted suicide* is widely disputed. Singer and Siegler (1990) present a summary of both sides of the case for and against euthanasia, though these authors are ethically and professionally against physician intervention in patient death. Doctors Quill (1990), and Cassel and Meier (1990) present another case for physician assisted suicide.

It is acknowledged that physicians on both sides of the argument may be ethical, well-meaning and mindful of their obligations to their patients. The point of differentiation seems to be what is referred to in bioethical terms as the "slippery slope." Simply defined, this term refers to the opinion that once intervention results in assisting death by any means, abuses and mistakes will multiply and before long, involuntary euthanasia may become wide spread. Another fear is the methodical elimination of burdens on society, such as the disabled, the incompetent, the elderly and other vulnerable groups. Opponents are also concerned that if physician assisted death becomes the norm, comfort care (i.e., hospice) and pain management will not be explored. The question opponents to euthanasia ask is: Can life be sacred if we take it upon ourselves to end a life?

Proponents of physician-assisted death cite the Netherlands experience where euthanasia is part of public policy and is circumscribed by explicit guidelines, requiring a clear and repeated request from the patient that leaves no uncertainly about the patient's competency and wish to die. Using the Netherlands' guidelines as a beacon, Dr. Timothy Quill has proposed his own clinical criteria for physician assisted suicide, but he distinguishes between assisted suicide which he supports, and active euthanasia which he does not support (Quill et al., 1992). Those on this side of the controversy

---

* For the purpose of this discussion, assisted death will be used for euthanasia and assisted suicide. But for clarity, *active euthanasia* is defined as the deliberate action by a physician to terminate life. In *assisted suicide* the physician prescribes but does not administer a lethal dose of medication.

feel that physicians should have the intellectual and moral vitality to stand by patients through the whole of life's course, including death. Proponents of euthanasia are also concerned that, in the absence of clearly defined ethical stances or public policies on assisted voluntary deaths, there may be more abuses and idiosyncratic decision-making than with a more open, carefully defined practice (Quill, 1992). In addition, if this process remains largely covert and unstudied, little will be known about which methods are most humane and effective, thereby denying patients the most pain-free death.

The concerns about euthanasia increase as we review the faith of the incompetent or unconscious person. As stated above, in New York and New Jersey differences about surrogate decision making could be a matter of where the ambulance takes the commuting accident victim; in New York he/she could remain in a vegetative state forever while in New Jersey, the family, in consultation with the physicians, can decide when to end the pain or the vegetative state. According to the latest decision by the U.S. Supreme Court in the Nancy Cruzan case (1990), "States have legitimate interest in preserving life regardless of its quality" (Annas, 1990, p. 670) therefore, the parent's request to have their daughter's feeding tube disconnected was refused despite the fact that she had been in a vegetative state for over seven years. Yet, in a poll conducted by Time/CNN after this court ruling, 80% of those surveyed felt decisions about ending the lives of terminally ill patients who cannot decide for themselves should be made by their families and physicians rather than lawmakers (Gibbs, 1990).

Ironically, the day the Supreme Court decided that Missouri (Cruzan v. Missouri) could "legitimately and rationally" assume that all families of incompetent patients could be a danger to them, it also decided that Ohio could "legitimately and rationally" assume that all families are loving and supportive and thus require a pregnant teenager to notify her parents before obtaining an abortion in order to uphold "the dignity of the family" (Ohio v. Akron Center for Reproductive Health, 1990). Consistent moral reasoning is not always evident in legal decision-making. When patients have no family or when family members cannot or will not agree about decisions, these conflicts will become society's burden, and laws may then become more defined.

A response to opponents of euthanasia's question asked earlier about the sanctity of life–can life be sacred if we take it upon ourselves to end a life?–could be the recognition that society often views giving up one's life as noble and self-sacrificing; in fact, we usually call these people "heroes." For many, the spiritual meaning of life creates a context in which death is not the enemy. Rather death is in fact sometimes to be welcomed as an appropriate and timely end to either a life fully lived or to a life cut short by the ravages of incurable disease (Cassel and Meier, 1990).

Both sides of this controversy emphasize that no decision about any clinical intervention should be made without a meaningful physician-patient relationship. This is especially true in making a final life decision. If euthanasia is to be performed, it must be in a very public manner where everyone involved is clear about their responsibilities and intentions, the procedural requirements are met, and there are people present to help the patient die with support and dignity.

SOCIETY'S PREDICAMENT

In the interviews reported in the Background section, several people were asked to react to the journal of a dying woman. The chief executive of a hospital, when asked who decides about life-ending choices, stated, in part, "society." This opinion can be viewed as honest and courageous. Without clarification of the legal and social status of physician assisted deaths by society, the physician and the hospitals remain vulnerable. As demonstrated above in the Supreme Court cases for the states of Missouri and Ohio, society's laws and policies offer conflicting messages about the country's willingness to support family rights. If society supports these Court decisions, then society should have to take a greater share of the responsibility, both ethically and morally, for life-ending decisions.

The precedent for sanctioning family rights over that of adult members is weakening, and the President's Commission on the Study of Ethical Problems recognized that family decision making must be kept within limits (President's Commission, 1983). In addition to recognizing that some patients have no families or that not all family members are supportive, there may be instances of families misusing their rights over the patient's because of the concern and stress involved in life threatening decisions (Lee and Berry, 1991).

Should society make decisions on life-ending choices based on economic or social concerns? How can we justify a high infant mortality rate as well as a public health care system that is in shambles while we spend tens of thousands of dollars a year to keep elderly, unconscious or incompetent patients alive (Gibbs, 1990)? How can we justify an increase in health care costs, which includes prolonging life through medical technology while thousands remain homeless? It is obvious that these and other questions will have to be debated with primary concern for the patient's comfort and care. These issues deserve a thorough and thoughtful analysis. The need for candid dialogue among physicians, attorneys, hospital administrators, bioethicists, patients and families is evident.

PATIENT RESPONSIBILITIES
AND FAMILY OBLIGATIONS

Several thoughts on patient responsibilities and family obligations are presented here. The conclusions are a synthesis of the exchanges of the persons interviewed about the content in the woman's journal.

The patient. Society currently has at its disposal many options for making adequate decisions for end of life. Each person may execute advance directives before needed; included in these directives–a living will that details as much as possible how to be treated if incompetent for any reason. This document could be as specific as possible and cover such interventions as tube feedings, respirators, resuscitation, medications, and so on. The patient's physician could help with a more inclusive list. Patients may opt for medical care as in a hospice model (referred to as comfort care), or as an alternative to traditional high technological intervention.

Individuals may appoint a proxy decision-maker with a durable power of attorney which is as limited as the patient deems necessary. Usually in a power of attorney for advance directives, decisions are limited to health and medical care only. Though the federal government enacted the Patient Self-Determination Act in 1991, the administrative and clinical barriers to having patients' advance directives honored still exist. A proxy designee to make medical decisions may be more effective than living wills; however, this is no guarantee. For this reason, advance directives, though important documents, are not substitutes for advanced planning with the patient's physician and family.

The best assurance one can have to maintain personal choice, if no extraordinary measures are requested, is to stay out of the hospital. As the caregiver stated in her interview, "If I want to make my own life-ending decisions, I wouldn't go to the hospital."

The family. Many believe that the family's primary duty is to honor the patient's wishes. The patient's wishes may be contrary to family members' values and morals. It may be difficult to stand by and "do nothing." However, it is important to remember that comfort care in a supportive atmosphere is a great deal more than "doing nothing." Remaining inactive may be the most difficult thing family members have to do, i.e., not dial 911, not phone for an ambulance, and not take the patient to the hospital. As the women said in her journal, "doing what is wrong for the right reasons, can never be right."

If there is a major dispute between the patient and the family about how to proceed, others outside the family unit may need to be involved, such as clergy or a therapist, depending on the patient's and the family's value system. However, the family's decision should not override that of the patient, unless the family determines that the patient is being coerced or made to feel guilty by others to make decisions inconsistent with his/her previously stated values.

DISCUSSION AND CONCLUSION

Ethical considerations in decision-making are multifaceted and complex. No one strategy, particularly in life/death choices, will respond to every situation, every need, every person. The woman whose journal was quoted in the beginning of the article might have been ready to die because she was depressed and disconnected from family, or she may have been in excruciating pain from the cancer. Her physician and the medical staff had an ethical obligation to treat the whole person and not merely the disease. Full treatment would have included psychotherapy for her depression, connection with a support group or community organization, physical pain relief, and perhaps a hospice-like setting to provide the support and comfort she needed and deserved. She could have been answered on all levels–physical, emotional and spiritual. The patient's request to die may signal the opportunity to discuss choices.

Dying is a part of living, and therefore, decisions about death are part of life decisions. Physician assisted suicide or euthanasia are ethical issues within the medical professions, but accountability must go beyond medical personnel. Society must also be answerable. Patients need to take responsibility and be active participants in their life and death decisions. Lay persons and professionals, working together, can bring about change through public and professional education. A society that proclaims to be humane cannot abandon those it alleges to be protecting: those mentally or physically impaired, the young, the aging and the disadvantaged.

Many find Dr. Jack Kevorkian's actions (active assisted suicide) detestable, but what about his intentions? Is he not shining a light on a dark and secretive issue and demanding that society respond by challenging the law and the courts? Changes in professional and personal ethics and values do not come easily nor are they without sacrifices. However, we need pioneers, not crusaders, and pioneers do not have road maps. Who decides? In one way or another, we all do.

REFERENCES

Annas, G.J. (1990). Nancy Cruzan and the right to die. *The New England J. of Medicine*, 323(10):670-673.

Caralis, P.V., Davis, B., Wright, K. and Marcial, E. (1993). The influence of ethnicity and race on attitudes towards advance directives, life-prolonging treatments and euthanasia. *The J. of Clin. Ethics*, 4(2):155-165.

Cassel, C.K. and Meier, D.E. (1990). Morals and moralism in the debate over euthanasia and assisted suicide. *The New England J. of Medicine*, 323(11): 750-752.

Cruzan v Director, Missouri Dept. of Health, 110 S.Ct 2841, 1990.

Emanuel, L. (1993). Advance directives: What have we learned so far? *The J. of Clin. Ethics*, 4(1):8-15.

Gibbs, N. (1990). Love and let die. *Time*, March 19:62-71.

Lee, M.A. and Berry, K. (1991). Abuse of durable power of attorney for health care: A case report. *J. Am. Geriatric Soc*, 39:806-809.

Ohio v Akron Center for Reproductive Health, 110 S.Ct 2972, 1990.

President's Commission for the Study of Ethical Problems in Medicine and Biomedical and Behavioral Research. (1983). Deciding to forgo life-sustaining treatment. Washington, DC: U.S. Govt. Printing Office, Chap. 4.

Quill, T.E. (1991). Death and dignity. *The New England J. of Medicine*, 324(10): 691-694.

Quill, T.E., Cassel, C.K. and Meier, D.E. (1992). Care of the hopelessly ill. *The New England J. of Medicine*, 327(19):1380-1384.

Singer, P.A. and Siegler, M. (1990). Euthanasia–A critique. *The New England J. of Medicine*, 322(26):1881-1883.

Supporting End of Life Decision Making

Linda L. Barrett

Each of us makes many decisions every day. Some of our choices have limited impact while other choices are felt more broadly. Similarly, our choices may be planned or occur by default. While taking a "wait and see" attitude may provide space for generating alternative solutions, denying problems or delaying decisions may limit the potential for creative problem solving. Creative problem solving, on the other hand, enables participants to craft solutions which everyone can accept. Basic principles can provide a useful foundation for shaping the decision-making process. The purpose of this article is to review end of life decision making among older adults in light of the basic principles of autonomy, non-maleficence and beneficence. Secondly, suggestions are presented for helping individuals, families and staff address these issues before a precipitating event requires unplanned actions to manage an unanticipated situation.

As the population ages, a growing number of older people face decisions concerning whether or not to receive life-sustaining medical treatments or to forgo treatment at the end of life. Until recently, little research focused directly on patients' choices concerning life sustaining treatments (High, 1988; High, 1990). One study, however, found that among hospital patients 64 to 97 years of age, 66% were

Linda L. Barrett, PhD, is Senior Research Associate, AARP Andrus Foundation, Washington, DC 20049. She has extensive expertise in planning and implementing programs on bioethics and end of life decision making for older adults.

[Haworth co-indexing entry note]: "Supporting End of Life Decision Making." Barrett, Linda L. Co-published simultaneously in *Activities, Adaptation & Aging* (The Haworth Press, Inc.) Vol. 18, No. 3/4, 1994, pp. 77-88; and: *Ethics and Values in Long Term Health Care* (ed: Patricia J. Villani) The Haworth Press, Inc., 1994, pp. 77-88. Multiple copies of this article/chapter may be purchased from The Haworth Document Delivery Center [1-800-3-HAWORTH; 9:00 a.m. - 5:00 p.m. (EST)].

more likely to want life sustaining treatments if they anticipated having cognitive capacity than if they anticipated cognitive impairment. Overall, these patients indicated their personal preferences for medical treatment were influenced most by their values, religion and experience with others illnesses (Cohen-Mansfield, 1992). Despite this, another study found that one third of the nurses who work in long term care settings in the United States, Canada and Australia report that physicians rarely, if ever, talk with their patients about their prognosis or treatment options. "Many nurses fear that clinical judgments about residents' care and their own values about quality of life and dignified death are overshadowed by fears of liability" (Lund, 1990: 223). On the other hand, obtaining informed consent may be viewed by health care providers as a way of avoiding malpractice suits (Hirsh, 1992; Kraushar, 1992).

In addition to safeguarding the medical profession, obtaining informed consent protects individual autonomy. Autonomy refers to honoring the right of individuals to make their own decisions. One of the most common applications of this principle in medicine is the mandate that health care providers obtain informed consent before implementing or withholding treatment. Hence, the argument for telling patients the truth about their health is based upon the belief that individual autonomy is critical in medical decision-making. Studies demonstrate that obtaining informed consent to provide a health care treatment is a process which occurs over time (Tymchuk, 1992). This process includes input, assimilation and decision phases. Hence, the individual obtains information and evaluates it in light of his/her values and beliefs before making decisions.

The issue of health care decision making with the informed consent of competent adults is relatively simple compared to situations when the adult is physically or mentally unable to consider, decide upon, and express his/her wishes. If adults routinely completed health care treatment directives, these written documents could convey patients' choices to others when they are unable to speak for themselves. Studies show, however, that only 4% to 18% of Americans 18 years of age or older have completed some form of advance directive (Society for the Right to Die, 1987; Wall Street Journal, 1988; Zweibel and Cassel, 1989). Thus, a majority of Americans have not documented their health care treatment preferences. At the same time, declining decisional capacity among the elderly is one of the most common issues health care professionals face when trying to obtain informed consent for treatment. Likewise, informed refusal of treatment is equally problematic for patients as they grow older and begin to lose decisional capacity.

Although there has been a reluctance to document treatment preferences in writing, studies have begun to examine older persons' preferences and expectations regarding health care decision-making following their loss of decisional capacity. Older people expect their family members to make decisions regarding their health care treatment when they are unable to express their choice (Shawler et al., 1992). (High, 1988, 1990) discovered that the lack of family was the primary reason for designating a health care proxy. Trusting the family, on the other hand, was the dominant reason for not wishing to appoint a proxy. High asserts that, close family surrogates are perceived by older adults to be naturally empowered by the autonomy accorded to the family unit and the family unit is the context in which individual autonomy arises and has its grounding (High and Turner, 1987).

When family members act as surrogates, one of two standards are applied for making decisions on behalf of older adults who have lost decisional capacity. These standards are substituted judgment and best interest. Both standards attempt to create decisions which are beneficial for the patient. Substituted judgment invites the proxy decision-maker to make the decision he/she believes the incapacitated patient would choose. The best interest standard invites the proxy to make a choice that he/she believes would be in the patient's best interest. While Jecker (1990) believes that caregivers develop intuitive knowledge about the wishes of the people they care for, many question whether or not family members are the most appropriate decision-makers for elderly incompetent patients by virtue of their relationship to the patient (High, 1990). In addition, studies demonstrate that family members and surrogates often do not agree with what the person would choose for him/herself (Butchelor et al., 1992; Hare et al., 1992). On the other hand, Tomlinson et al., (1990) found that when related subjects were explicitly asked to make a substituted judgment they came significantly closer to the elderly person's preferences than those who were asked to make their best choice recommendation.

Regardless of one's position on the involvement of family members, physicians usually seek family members' consent when deciding on treatment for elderly incompetent patients (Sherlock and Dingus, 1985). One of the most challenging situations is dealing with Alzheimer disease patients. Patients who have Alzheimer's disease are on a "path of declining capacity to give consent, (and) advancement of research with Alzheimer's disease subjects present challenging and perplexing ethical and legal dilemmas" (High, 1992). It is important to note, however, that Alzheimer's disease is not the only form of mental incapacity. At least one study (Wear, 1991) has shown that health professionals may want to override the decisions made by patients who have a mental disorder even though having a mental illness does not necessarily mean he/she is unable to make such decisions for him/herself.

Even in situations where a dying patient is competent, Slomka (1992) acknowledges that clinical decisions involve people (dying patients, physicians and their families) who may bring different perceptions and interpretations to the decision-making process. Hence death becomes a negotiated process and the philosophical principles which seem clear in theory become blurred in application. For example ethicists view the withholding and withdrawing of life-supporting treatments as morally equivalent. However, " . . . physicians tend to make a distinction based on the perceived locus of moral responsibility for the patient's death" (Slomka, 1992). Slomka (1992) interprets "the moral responsibility for the patient's death by withdrawing treatment is shared with family members, while the moral responsibility for the patient's death by withholding treatment is displaced to the patient." He suggests that there is an illusion of choice in the medical decision-making physicians offer patients and that the negotiation of meaning creates a shared moral responsibility for medical failure and its eventual acceptance by patient, family and physician. Here again, there may be times when parties do not agree about the course of action and there is some question about whether it is justified to withdraw life support against the family's wishes (Edwards, 1988) or whether patients are entitled to futile treatment (Gold et al., 1989). Hence making decisions in medical situations can be difficult when participants bring different perceptions and/or expectations to the process or when adherence to one philosophical principle clashes with another.

Two emerging issues highlight acts which may hinder or hasten death and thus emphasize the important relationship between the patient and his/her health care providers. The first issue concerns the interpretation and implementation of do not resuscitate orders (DNR) and the second addresses the issue of assisted suicide. While implementing physicians' medical orders may appear straightforward, investigations show that an interpretative process occurs which can influence life and death decisions (Enderlin and Wilhite, 1991; Murphy, 1990; Ventres et al., 1992). The interpretation of DNR orders reflect cultural and professional values, previous personal experience and providers' assumptions (Ventres, 1992). These orders may be interpreted literally or quite broadly (Murphy, 1990). When DNRs are interpreted literally, staff will not implement cardiopulmonary resuscitation (CPR) when the patient's heart stops functioning yet will provide other treatments. On the other hand, if DNR orders are interpreted broadly, staff may withdraw all medical treatments and only provide palliative care. Consequently, older people may be at risk for receiving inadequate care (Murphy, 1990; Kern, 1992).

The second act takes health care providers another step toward hastening death. Physician assisted suicide and euthanasia are highly controversial issues. Although suicide is not typically considered an illegal act, helping another to commit suicide is considered to be a crime in most states. Even so, a public opinion poll reported that a majority of Americans favor the idea of medically assisted suicide for terminally ill patients (Newsweek, 1990). In addition, Derek Humphrey, executive director of the Hemlock Society, wrote a book entitled *Final Exit* that supported the idea that suicide and assisted suicide are rational acts when one is facing the unbearable suffering of terminal illness. The popularity of Humphrey's book indicates some people desire information and/or help dealing with the possibility of ending their life.

Two empirical studies have investigated these issues. Watts et al. (1992) studied geriatricians attitudes toward assisting in demented patients' suicide with specific reference to the case of Janet Adkins.

Mrs. Adkins was diagnosed with Alzheimer's disease and was assisted in committing suicide by Jack Kevorkian, MD. The findings showed that 14% of the 727 geriatricians surveyed in this study believed Dr. Kevorkian's assistance was morally justifiable. Sixty-six percent did not think his assistance was justifiable and the remaining 20% were unsure. Those who opposed the act frequently cited the principle and oath of doing no harm (non-maleficence) to support their view. While 29% thought the act was morally wrong, 49% did not think it was morally wrong. These geriatricians also reported that if they were personally diagnosed with a dementing illness 41% would consider suicide, 39% would not consider suicide. In addition over one quarter of these physicians favored easing the restrictions on physician assisted suicide while 57% opposed easing these restrictions. Physician attitudes varied by geographic location with the Midwestern region exhibiting the most conservative physician attitudes.

The second study (Hiller and Sugarman, 1990) examined the attitudes of 193 long term care professionals toward assisted suicide and euthanasia under specific situations. The majority of respondents, 76.2%, thought that terminally ill residents should have the right to end their lives. They did not think it was acceptable to maintain a resident on life support if the resident had completed an advance directive. These respondents consistently emphasized the important role physicians play in determining residents' competency to make such decisions. Despite these observations, they were ambivalent about the use of physician assisted suicide machines.

While clinical issues are important in long term care settings, everyday issues are important to residents. This includes having a choice about what, where and when to eat. Choosing what to wear, who one's roommate will be, how to protect one's privacy and whether or not to participate in structured activities are also autonomy issues. Having the right to personal property, including the expectancy of receiving your own clothes back from the laundry, are important personal security issues. While these may appear insignificant from a clinical perspective, from the resident's perspective these are the issues which significantly influence the quality of life in long term care (Kaplan, 1990).

In summary, we know: (1) most people have not documented

their health care treatment preferences in the event they can not communicate their wishes, (2) physicians frequently turn to families to help make treatment decisions when the patient is unable to decide for him/herself, (3) families may, or may not, be able to make decisions that reflect the patients'/residents' choice, (4) the typical long term care resident is an older widow who has several chronic health conditions and functional losses (Kane and Kane, 1982), (5) a large proportion of long term care residents have some degree of mental incapacity and (6) adult children may find themselves making choices which they are unprepared to make. Given these conditions, several investigators (Kaplan, 1990; Moody, 1992) have questioned the usefulness of applying the concept of autonomy to long term care residents as one might to a younger acute care patient. Most agree that a continuum of autonomy can help bridge the gap between those residents who may be able to participate in decision making and those are unprepared to participate. Therefore, a variety of people, including residents, family, physicians and long term care staff, may have differing degrees of involvement in the decision making process depending upon the residents' mental and physical capacity. Consequently, it is important for significant others to be involved as early as possible in discussions about end of life treatment and quality of life preferences.

When I managed community based health information programs between 1989 and 1992 more community dwelling older adults chose to attend our programs on advance directives than any other health related issue. Our purpose was to provide accurate and timely information on how to complete health care treatment directives such as a living will and durable power of attorney for health care. Equally important was encouraging participants to discuss their wishes with significant others such as family, physician, attorney, minister or priest, friends, financial planner. We consistently found participants were eager for information and were willing to engage their significant others in discussions about these issues.

As the literature review demonstrates, however, a majority of Americans have not completed health care treatment directives. Therefore, the process of planning for end of life decisions may be facilitated in long term care settings by the Patient Self Determination Act of 1990. This Act was part of the Omnibus Budget Reconciliation Act of 1990 and is commonly referred to as the Patient Self Determination Act (PSDA). This Act, which went into effect on December 1, 1991, requires health care providers to inform patients about their rights to execute advance directives such as living wills and durable powers of attorney for health care. It specifically requires all hospitals, nursing facilities, home health care agencies, hospices, and health maintenance organizations participating in the Medicare and Medicaid programs provide written materials on advance directives to all adults who come to them as patients. These providers are also required to inform people of their rights under state law to make health care choices. This means that providers need to know their state laws, document and implement institutional policies regarding the PSDA, identify and train staff who will be responsible for providing patient education as well as collecting information and regularly auditing organizational compliance with PSDA requirements.

While each facility is required to develop its own plan to implement the PSDA, there are numerous ways to kindle the spirit of the law as well as the letter of the law. In addition to informing patients about their rights to create health care treatment directives, a supportive environment can be created which encourages residents, family and staff to explore difficult issues before a crisis emerges. This environment can: (1) encourage open communication between providers, families and residents about treatment decisions, how these decisions will be implemented, and everyday quality of life issues, (2) provide time and space for families and residents to contemplate choices and (3) help providers, families and residents resolve their differences of opinion and help individuals resolve their internal conflicts. Long term care staff can work cooperatively to help facilitate these processes by developing a formal plan mandated by the PSDA. In addition, community based volunteer programs can be replicated in long term care facilities. Support in planning and implementing these sessions can come from community, or university-based ethics centers, health decision centers, or local medical and/or bar associations. Panel presentations create an opportunity to share the views of religious leaders, medical, nursing, legal and financial professions. Panels are especially effective when questions and answers are encouraged from the audience. The audience can be a mixture of residents, family and staff. The Health Advocacy Services section of AARP currently offers a no, or low cost program entitled "Who Decides When You Can't? Planning Family Medical Decisionmaking" which focuses on the family unit. Your institution may also consider forming a long term care ethics committee to help formulate policy and support the decision making process. Coming to terms with end of life issues is not an easy process; however, recognizing choices and planning for change provides a sense of control which is lost when decisions are made by default. Perhaps if we assume our responsibility for helping make these choices and for creating a health and long term care system which addresses peoples' needs, we can avoid the desire felt by some to resort to assisted suicide.

REFERENCES

American Association of Retired Persons, Health Advocacy Services, (1993). Who Decides When You Can't? Planning Family Medical Decisionmaking. Washington, DC.

Areen, J. (1987). The Legal Status of Consent Obtained from Families of Adult Patients to Withhold or Withdraw Treatment. *JAMA*, 258, 229-235.

Batchelor, A. J. et al. (1992). Predictors of Advance Directives Restrictiveness and Compliance with Institutional Policy in a Long-Term Care Facility. *Journal of the American Geriatrics Society*, 7: 679-684.

Beck, M. (1990). Doctor's Suicide Van. *Newsweek*, 115: 46-47.

Callahan, D. (1987). Setting Limits: Medical Goals in an Aging Society. New York, NY: Simon & Schuster.

Callahan, D. (1992). Limiting Health Care for the Old. In. N. S. Jecker (Ed.) Aging and Ethics (pp. 219-226). Clifton, NJ: Humana Press.

Callahan, M. R. (1991). Prepping for Patient Self-Determination Act. *Modern Healthcare*, 21: 36.

Caplan, Arthur L. (1990). The Morality of the Mundane: Ethical Issues Arising In The Daily Lives of Nursing Home Residents. In R. A. Kane and A. L. Caplan (Eds.), Everyday Ethics Resolving Dilemmas in Nursing Home Life (pp. 37-50). New York: Springer Publishing Company.

Capron, A. M. (1992). The Patient Self-Determination Act: New Responsibilities for Health Care Providers. *Journal of American Health Policy*, 2: 40-43.

Cohen-Mansfield, J. et al. (1992). Factors Influencing Hospital Patients' Preferences in the Utilization of Life-Sustaining Treatments. *Gerontologist*, 32: 89-95.

Daniels, N. (1992). A Lifespan Approach to Health Care. In N. S. Jecker (Ed.), Aging and Ethics (pp. 222-246). Clifton, NJ: Humana Press.

Dautzenberg, P. L and P. D. Bezemer (1991). Quantitative and Qualitative Aspects of Cardiopulmonary Resuscitation in Aged In-Patients. *Netherlands Journal of Medicine*, 39: 366-372.

Deimling, G. et al. (1990). Health Care Professionals and Family Involvement in Care-Related Decisions Concerning Older Patients. *Journal of Aging and Health*, 2, 310-325.

Drickamer, M. A. and M. S. Lachs. (1992). Should patients with Alzheimer's disease be told their diagnosis? *New England Journal of Medicine*, 326: 947-951.

Edwards, B. S. (1990). Withdrawal of Life Support Against Family Wishes: Is It Justified? A Case Study. *Journal of Clinical Ethics*, 1: 74-79.

Gibson, J. M. (1990). National Values History Project. In Generations Supplement 1990 on Autonomy and Long-Term Care.

Gibson, J. M. (1991). Advance Directives in the 1990s. Paper available from the Center for Health Law and Ethics, Institute of Public Law.

Gold, J. A. (1990). Is There a Right to Futile Treatment? The Case of a Dying Patient with AIDS. *Journal of Clinical Ethics*, 1:19-23.

Hare, J. et al. (1992). Agreement Between Patients and Their Self-Selected Surrogates on Difficult Medical Decisions. *Archives of Internal Medicine*, 152: 1049-1054.

Henderson, M. (1990). Beyond the Living Will. *Gerontologist*, 30, 480-485.

High, D. (1987). Surrogate Decision-Making: The Elderly's familial expectations. *Theoretical Medicine*, 8, 303-320.

High, D. (1988). All in the Family: Extended Autonomy and Expectations in Surrogate Health Care Decision-Making. *Gerontologist*, 28, 46-51.

High, D. (1992). Research with Alzheimer's Disease Subjects: Informed Consent with Proxy Decision Making. *Journal of the American Geriatrics Society*, 40: 950-957.

High, D. (1990). Who Will Make Health Care Decisions for Me When I Can't? *Journal of Aging and Health*, 2, 291-309.

High, D. (1990). Old and Alone: Surrogate Health Care Decision-Making for the Elderly Without Families. *Journal of Aging Studies*, 4: 277-288.

Hiller, M.D. and D.B. Sugarman. (1990). Euthanasia and Long-Term Care: Values of the Long-Term Care Professional. *Journal of Long-Term Care Administration*, 18: 23-30.

Hirsch, B. D. (1992). Avoiding Malpractice Claims for Lack of Informed Consent. *Medical Staff Counsel*. 6: 57-65.

Jecker, N. S. (1990). The Role of Intimate Others in Medical Decision Making. *Gerontologist*, 30, 65-71.

Jecker, N. S. (1992). Aging and Ethics. Clifton, NJ: Humana Press.

Kane, R. L. and R. A. Kane (1982). Values and Long-Term Care. Lexington, MA: Lexington Books.

Kayser-Jones, J. (1990). The Use of Nasogastric Feeding Tubes in Nursing Homes: Patient, Family and Health Care Provider Perspectives. *Gerontologist*, 30, 469-479.

Kern, D. et al. (1992). Do-Not-Resuscitate Order for Patients Undergoing Bone Marrow Transplantation. *Oncology Nurses Forum*, 19: 635-640.

Kraushar, M. F. (1992). Recognizing and Managing the Litigious Patient. *Surv Ophtalmol*, 37: 54-56.

Lamm, R. The Aging Connection 9, 10. 10, 10.

LaPuma, J. et al. (1991). Advance Directives on Admission: Clinical Implications and Analysis of the Patient Self-Determination Act of 1990. *JAMA*, 266: 402-405

Lipsky, M. S. (1989). DNR orders: Helping your patients decide. *Senior Patient*, May/June 77-80.

Lund, M. (1990). Speaking Out on Ethics. *Geriatric Nursing*, 11: 223-227.

Lurie, Nicole et al. (1992). Attitudes Toward Discussing Life-Sustaining Treatments In Extended Care Facility Patients. *Journal of the American Geriatrics Society*, 12: 1205-1208.

Malloy, T. R. et al. (1992). Influence of Treatment Descriptions on Advance Medical Directive Decisions. *Journal of the American Geriatrics Society*, 40: 1255-1260.

McCullough, L. B. (1992). Ethical Issues Related to Technology in the Care of Hospitalized Elderly Patients: The Primacy of Preventive Ethics. *International Journal of Technology and Aging*, 5: 187-194.

Moody, H. R. (1992). The Meaning of Life in Old Age. In N. S. Jecker, (Ed.), Aging and Ethics. Clifton, NJ: Humana Press.

Moody, H. R. (1992). Ethics in an Aging Society. Baltimore, MD: Johns Hopkins University Press.

Moss, R. J. and J. La Puma (1991). Ethics of Mechanical Restraints. *Hastings Center Report*, 21: 22-25.

Murphy, D. J. (1990). Improving Advance Directives for Healthy Older People. *Journal of the American Geriatrics Society*, 38: 1251-1256.

Orentlicher, D. (1992). The Illusion of Patient Choice in End-of-Life Decisions. *JAMA*, 267: 2101-2104.

Rawls, J. (1971). A Theory of Justice. Cambridge, MA: Harvard University Press.

Shawler, C. et al. (1992). Clinical Considerations: Surrogate Decision Making for Hospitalized Elders. *Journal of Gerontological Nursing*, 18: 5-11.

Sherlock, R. and M. Dingus (1985). Families and the Gravely Ill: Roles, Rules and Rights. *Journal of the American Geriatrics Society*, 33, 121-124.

Slomka, J. (1992). The Negotiation of Death: Clinical Decision Making at the End of Life. *Social Science Medicine*, 35: 251-259.

Society for the Right to Die. (1987). Newsletter, Spring.

Terrenoire, G. (1992). Huntington's Disease and the Ethics of Genetic Prediction. *Journal of Medical Ethics*, 18: 79-85.

Tomlinson, T. et al. (1990). An Empirical Study of Proxy Consent for Elderly Persons. *Gerontologist*, 30, 55-64.

Tymchuk, A. J. and J. G. Ouslander (1990). Optimizing the Informed Consent Process with Elderly People. *Educational Gerontology*, 16, 245-257.

Tymchuk, A. J. and J. G. Ouslander (1992). Alternative conceptualization of informed consent with people who are elderly. *Educational Gerontology,* 18:135-147.

Ventres, W. et al. (1992). Do-Not-Resuscitate Discussions: A Qualitative Analysis. *Family Practice Resident Journal,* 12: 157-169.

Watts, D. T. , T. Howell and B. A. Priefer (1992). Geriatricians' attitudes toward assisting suicide of dementia patients. *Journal of the American Geriatrics Society,* 40: 878-885.

Waymack, M. H. (1992). Old Age and the Rationing of Scarce Health Care Resources. In N. S. Jecker (Ed.), Aging and Ethics. (pp. 247-267). Clifton, NJ: Humana Press.

Wear, A. N. and D. Brahams (1991). To Treat or Not to Treat: The Legal, Ethical and Therapeutic Implications of Treatment Refusal. *Journal of Medical Ethics,* 17: 131-135.

Zweibel, N. R. and Cassel, C. K. (1989). Treatment choices at the end of life: A Comparison of decisions by older patients and their physician-selected proxies. *Gerontologist,* 29, 615-621.

The Ethical Value of a Utilitarian Approach to Death and Dying

Vera R. Jackson

BACKGROUND

Many care providers are often uncomfortable with the task of enabling the aged to plan for their death. Researchers are equally uncomfortable with the task of delving into the realms of death and dying with this population because of societal expectations. There is an implicit expectation that the old will die before the young (Franke & Durlak, 1990; Rando, 1985). We assume that the aged by virtue of chronological age have made provisions for death and are ready to accept the inevitability. However, as many aged persons fear death as the non-aged (Franke & Durkak, 1990; Missinne & Willeke-Kay, 1985).

As society indicates an increased willingness to face death, and researchers provide the necessary information to deal with its reality, there is reason to hope that ours may be one of the last generations reared in an abysmal ignorance of life's greatest certainty. Undoubtedly, there is the propensity for man to die reluctantly, but he can die in a manner consistent with the personal values by which he has lived.

Vera R. Jackson, PhD, is Executive Director, Junior Citizens Corps, Inc., and is affiliated with the George Washington University Department of Health and Human Services, Washington, DC.

[Haworth co-indexing entry note]: "The Ethical Value of a Utilitarian Approach to Death and Dying." Jackson, Vera R. Co-published simultaneously in Activities, Adaptation & Aging (The Haworth Press, Inc.) Vol. 18, No. 3/4, 1994, pp. 89-94; and: Ethics and Values in Long Term Health Care (ed: Patricia J. Villani) The Haworth Press, Inc., 1994, pp. 89-94. Multiple copies of this article/chapter may be purchased from The Haworth Document Delivery Center [1-800-3-HAWORTH; 9:00 a.m. - 5:00 p.m. (EST)].

SOCIETAL POLARITY

The problems associated with death are beginning to polarize at two different points within the social structure. The first area of concern is the disengagement of the aged from a society that is becoming less interested in them as individuals or as functionaries within the social system. The second difficulty is the excessive concern our society has for the young. Our American value system puts the aged in double jeopardy by indicating that "it is better to work than not" and "better to be young than old" (Missinne & Willeke-Kay, 1985).

The problems are further intensified by the fact that there is yet no empirical methods for demonstrating whether or not the patterns of behavior observed in attempting to cope with death are functionally relevant. According to Borkenau (1965), the conflicting attitudes toward death unconsciously experienced by the individual are also at work within the culture, so that ultimately there emerge periods when the culture can be characterized as "death denying" in outlook.

Goldscheider's (1978) article on "The Social Inequality of Death" reminds us that just as people do not have equal standards of living or incomes, neither does death confront us on an egalitarian basis. While most deaths today occur among the elderly, society offers the pretense that responses to death are both balanced and equal.

MORAL VS. TECHNICAL ORDERS

As society and culture changes, so do prevailing moral and ethical values. Death has come to be perceived as both a moral matter and a technical matter. The moral order has been used to describe those bonds between men, based on sentiment or conscience, that describe what is right. The technical order rests on the usefulness of things, based on necessity and expediency, and is not often founded in right versus wrong conceptualizations.

Moral and ethical terms that are sometimes used interchangeably do not refer to a preordained ideal or universal set of beliefs or actions. The statement that one's actions are guided by moral principles does not imply that these principles are inherently "good" or "proper" according to some higher standard or pre-existing design.

"Moral behavior involves more than simply the decisions and choices men make about specific problems; it also includes the kind of men they are (their character and virtues), the kind of beliefs they hold, and the way they integrate and organize their resources and energies to form a coherent life plan" (Hauerwas, 1974).

Moral conflicts may be as varied as human experiences themselves. When individuals take the time to reflect on troubling questions about morality, thoughts, and actions, they notice that different encounters evoke somewhat different demands on their abiding thoughts and feelings about what is good, right, obligatory, fair, and so on. The complexities of human relationships, the contingencies of living, and how people define themselves in different times and places may arouse certain variations in the most coherent and cherished set of moral beliefs or, for that matter, put these dependable beliefs in serious doubt.

It does not matter that the death of a person cannot be removed from the moral order by the very nature of personhood. What matters is the mythology of the society. The widespread mythology that things essentially moral can be made technical is reinforced by the effect of technology in altering other events besides death.

THE UTILITARIAN APPROACH

Research literature on the ethical aspects of death and dying tends to reflect segmental philosophies instead of a universal perspective which governs all regardless of medical or chronological status. Yet few researchers and practitioners move beyond the basic questions concerning meaning and method to questions based upon those principles by which all moral agents ought to be guided. A case in point is utilitarianism. The fundamental principle underlying the theory of utilitarianism is that acts are right if they bring the greatest possible balance of intrinsic good over intrinsic evil for everyone concerned, otherwise they are wrong.

Utilitarianism is an ethical theory that provides criterion for distinguishing between right and wrong action and an account of the nature of the moral judgements that characterize action as right or wrong. In its standard form, it can be expressed as the combination of two principles: (1) the consequentialist principle that the rightness or wrongness, of an action is determined by the goodness, or badness, of the results that flow from it and (2) the hedonist principle that the only thing that is good in itself is pleasure and the only thing bad in itself is pain. Utilitarians generally believe that happiness is a sum of pleasures.

Most often attributed to Jeremy Bentham, utilitarians believe that an "action is best which procures the greatest happiness of the greatest number" (Bentham, 1962). The simple core of the doctrine lies in the ideas that actions should be judged by their consequences and that the best actions are those which make people, as a whole, better off than do the alternatives.

Consider an illustration for understanding utilitarianism based upon the work of John Day (1990), and modified to encompass the disparities that exist in death and dying. A utilitarian might argue against a research investment which has as a focus policies and practices designed to help the aged prepare for death and dying. Instead, the utilitarian would advocate for research on a younger population, based upon logic that the old have less time to live than the young and therefore are less likely to benefit from this research effort. While the aged are as much entitled as the nonaged to the benefits of this research focus on death and dying, the utilitarian would calculate the amount of relief against the distress and would make the decision that the non-aged should be the focus of this research consideration.

Whose satisfaction should be promoted when the interests of different people and groups come into conflict? In theory, utilitarianism can always decide which is the right course of action by calculating what maximizes utility, whether this is interpreted as the balance of pleasure and pain or the weighing of individual's preferences. The theory seems fair in that it treats all individuals affected by an action as equally important. However, the practicalities of calculating utility are often at least as problematical as those produced by trying to decide priorities by comparing needs and the ends to which they are relevant.

The utilitarian weighs the good resulting from a particular action on the community as a whole. So an action would be justified on utilitarian grounds if it achieved the best possible balance between distress and relief even if the greatly increased benefit to the vast majority entailed the total neglect of a suffering minority.

In application, most of the planning we currently see in this country for the aged is based upon utilitarian ethics. We consider most often what is best for the larger good which is consistently composed of non-aged persons over the general welfare of the aged.

THE ALL INCLUSIVE MODEL

How, then, do we move from the driving force of utilitarianism ethics towards theories, models, principles and practices that encompasses death and dying for all regardless of chronological age? First, there must be a theoretical acknowledgement of death as an event and dying as a process. Second, there must occur an acknowledgement of the universality of death. Finally, a consensus must occur among researchers and practitioners that some form of model must be considered utilizing the positive qualities of utilitarianism. This model must be an ethical, valid, and appropriate framework for application.

One such model that could serve as a practical guide to action must at a minimum encompass the following elements:

1. A strong regard for humanity.
2. A specified methodology that includes distributional criteria. At a basic minimum, all people would have to be entitled to the same basic standards.
3. Research, policy, and application opportunities that are available to all people rather than on the basis of the use they make of these opportunities.
4. Personal freedom that is emphasized as a tenet of choice. In other words, all people must have the enhanced opportunities for choice and expression of personal preferences.

CONCLUSION

The belief is widespread that society's approach to death and dying is primarily embedded in a utilitarian ethical approach. Unfortunately, the aged tend to be weighed unfavorably in the balance when compared to the non-aged. Until efforts are made to either modify existing ethical theories to make them more universal for all, these disparities will continue. Further research will allow for the adaptation of theories and the development of a foundation of knowledge that will enhance death and dying education and provisions.

REFERENCES

Bentham, Jeremy. (1962). *The Works of Jeremy Bentham.* Vol. 1, pp. 142-143. New York: Russell and Russell.

Borkenau, Frank. (1965). The Concept of Death. In *Death and Identity.* R. Fulton (Ed.), page 46. New York, New York: John Wiley and Sons.

Day, John. (1990). Justice and Utility in Health Care. In *Utilitarian Response.* Pp. 30-56. Lincoln Allison (Ed.). London, England: Sage Publications.

Franke, Kevin J. & Durlak, Joseph A. Impact of Life Factors Upon Attitudes Toward Death. *Omega, 21*(1), 41-49.

Goldscheider, Calvin. (1978). The Social Inequality of Death. In *Death and Dying: Challenge and Change.* Fulton, Robert, et al. (Ed.). Regents of the University of California.

Hauerwas, S. (1974). *The Self as Story: A Reconsideration of the Relation of Religion and Morality from the Agents' Perspective Vision and Virtue Essays in Christian Ethical Consideration.* Pp. 68-69. Notre Dame, IN: Fids Publishing Company.

Missinne, Leo & Willeke-Kay, Judy. (1985, Summer) Reflections on the Meaning of Life in Older Age. *Journal of Religion & Aging.* Vol 1(4), pp. 43-58.

Rando, Therese A. (1985, Jan-Feb). Bereaved Parents: Particular Difficulties, Unique Factors, and Treatment Issues. *Social Work.* Vol 30 (1), pp. 19-23.

HEALTH CARE REFORM

Ethics and Health Care Reform: Outlook for Older Americans

Marie Raber
Michelle Hawkins

Health and social services for the older adult have evolved in this country without the benefit of systematic planning and goal setting (Monk, 1990). Services have resulted from public and political demands to meet the existing needs of the older adult. As a result, programs and services which have evolved are fragmented and ineffective in meeting the varying degree of health and social services needs of the older adult.

In response to emerging health care proposals, this article examines proposed services in relation to the stated principles and values as applied to the health care needs of elderly Americans. According to President Clinton's Health Care Proposal, certain values and principles are the underpinning of the entire proposal (Clinton Health Care Policy, 1993, p. 11). These are:

- *Universal Access:* Every American citizen and legal resident should have access to health care without financial or other barriers.

- *Comprehensive Benefits:* Guaranteed benefits should meet the full range of health needs, including primary, preventive and specialized care.

Marie Raber, DSW, is Assistant Dean, and Michelle Hawkins, PhD, is Assistant Professor National Catholic School of Social Service, Catholic University of America, Washington, DC.

[Haworth co-indexing entry note]: "Ethics and Health Care Reform: Outlook for Older Americans." Raber, Marie, and Michele Hawkins. Co-published simultaneously in *Activities, Adaptation & Aging* (The Haworth Press, Inc.) Vol. 18, No. 3/4, 1994, pp. 97-105; and: *Ethics and Values in Long Term Health Care* (ed: Patricia J. Villani) The Haworth Press, Inc., 1994, pp. 97-105. Multiple copies of this article/chapter may be purchased from The Haworth Document Delivery Center [1-800-3-HAWORTH; 9:00 a.m. - 5:00 p.m. (EST)].

- *Choice:* Each consumer should have the opportunity to exercise effective choice about providers, plans and treatments. Each consumer should be informed about what is known about the risks and benefits of available treatments and be free to choose among them according to his or her preferences.
- *Equality of Care:* The system should avoid the creation of a two tier system providing care based only on differences of need, not individualized or group characteristics.
- *Fair Distribution of Costs:* The health care system should spread the costs and burdens of care across the entire community, basing the level of contribution required of consumers on ability to pay.
- *Personal Responsibility:* Under health reform, each individual and family should assume responsibility for protecting and promoting health and contributing to the cost of care.
- *Intergenerational Justice:* The health care system should respond to the unique needs of each stage of life, sharing benefits and burdens fairly across generations.
- *Wise Allocation of Resources:* The nation should balance prudently what it spends on health care against other important national priorities.

It is imperative that these principles and values are reflected in any legislation for health care for our citizens. First, this article will examine these principles and values in relation to the current health care provisions for the elderly. Second, the Clinton Health Care Proposal will be analyzed to see if these principles and values are reflected in provisions for the elderly.

Universal Access. While Medicare is inadequate, this legislation has attempted to bring universal health care coverage to our elderly. Most U.S. citizens 65 and older are covered by Medicare Part A (hospitalization, limited nursing home care and institutional needs) and approximately 90% are enrolled in Part B (professional fees for medical and surgical services) (Stoline & Weiner, 1993). However, this legislation has proven less than adequate in many respects, especially due to the excessive number of rules and regulations.

The inordinate number of rules have made access particularly difficult for the elderly American. The need for deductibles, cost sharing and a variety of exclusions compounded this inequity by passing on significant costs to the elderly (Monk, 1990). Furthermore, Medicare has provided care for acute illness and hospital care, failing to provide reasonable access to prevention, rehabilitation and home care services. These factors present the major barriers to providing universal health care creating a two tier system for those elderly with financial means and those without.

In the President's current proposed legislation, The Medicare system would virtually remain the same. If the proposal is passed as written, persons currently enrolled in Medicare would remain. Persons turning 65 after the proposal is enacted would have the choice to join Medicare or remain in their current health care plan. Therefore, by leaving those currently in the plan, the lack of full coverage would remain for a significant number of our elderly.

Comprehensive Benefits. As stated previously, many benefits are not covered under Medicare. Along with the deductibles, exclusions and need for third party coverage, Medicare does not cover dental services and hearing devices, physician charges exceeding Medicare limits and extended stays at nursing homes. In fact, it is these uncovered nursing home costs and lack of coverage for prescription drugs that point to the inadequacy of benefits for the elderly. The lack of nursing home coverage has been a major obstacle to the elderly and their families, in some cases, causing financial and emotional disaster. Furthermore, with the rising costs of prescription drugs, many elderly have faced decisions of continuing their prescriptions or paying for other expenses such as food.

While the intended goal of Medicare was to provide needed health care for our elderly citizens, out-of-pocket expenses have rapidly increased, nearly doubling during the past 10 years (Stoline and Weiner, 1993). Unfortunately, Social Security benefits have not increased at a pace that would cover these rising costs. Therefore, out-of-pocket medical expenses are taking a higher percentage of the elderly's income.

Under the President's current proposal, two previously uncovered areas of need would be addressed. First, prescription drugs would be covered. The prescription drug coverage would be added to the cost of Medicare at a cost of $11 per month for persons covered in the Part B Medicare program. Furthermore, there would be a 20% co-payment with a $250 deductible, with an annual limit of $1,000 for out-of-pocket expenses. The prescription coverage would include insulin and other biological products.

Second, long term care needs are addressed in the proposal. Long term home care and/or community-based outpatient care would be provided for individuals needing assistance with three out of five of the following activities: eating, dressing, bathing, toileting or getting in and out of bed. However, nursing home care would be only slightly expanded by increasing Medicaid eligibility. Tax incentives for long-term care insurance would be added.

Choice of Providers. Persons covered by Medicare should have choice of providers, but in actuality, they do not. Not every physician accepts Medicare, and for those that do, their fees often exceed the limits of Medicare. What is worse is the attitude of many heath care practitioners who discourage Medicare patients who do not have the additional coverage or ability to "pay more" than the Medicare limits. The greatest barrier to choice of provider as well as comprehensive benefits for the elderly has been the increasingly large number of physicians, especially specialists, who refuse to honor the Medicare limits for those elderly who cannot pay their fees.

Along with the current health proposal, there have been suggestions to cut Medicare's projected growth over a five year period which would save $124 billion. This limit in growth, along with current barriers in the system, could have a negative impact on the number of physicians willing to accept Medicare patients. This added barrier could limit choices of physicians for the elderly. While advocating the need for every American to have freedom of choice in the selection of doctors, the current plan makes it obvious that many people will have to pay more for this choice. Some of the other proposed plans will require extra payment for physicians outside of these plans.

Equality of Care. Affluent Americans get better health care than less affluent, especially the elderly who depend on Medicare. This form of socioeconomic discrimination is what has led to present demand for health care reform in this country. Poor people get poor health care. Societal values, especially the underlying motives of many young adults entering our medical schools, has been the pursuit of wealth, not the well-being of society.

While equality of care is a definite concern in Clinton's Health Care Proposal, this equality seems to remain with those under 65 years of age. By continuing Medicare in it's current form while implementing another plan with different benefits for younger Americans, a two-tier system would result. For instance, in the current proposal, the standard package would have a limit on out-of-pocket expenses of $1,500 per year for individuals and $3,000 for families. Currently, Medicare recipients do not have overall limits on out-of-pocket costs. Furthermore, they must pay a deductible of $696 for the first 60 days of each hospitalization and increasing shares for stays past 60 days.

Another difference for the two systems is the pricing of premiums in relation to incomes. Currently, under Medicare, all recipients pay the same amount for premiums regardless of income. Under the current proposal, Medicare premiums would triple for individuals with incomes higher than $90,000 and $115,000 for families. However, for younger Americans, the amount of income would not determine the price of premiums. The inequality of a two-tier system has been a concern of AARP (American Association of Retired Persons) (AARP, November, 1993).

Fair Distribution of Costs. While there is a growing trend to have those who earn more to pay more for health care, reform has been slow with little grass roots support in the political arena or medical profession. Medicare and Medicaid cannot support the need for long term care for elderly Americans (Monk, 1991). With the Clinton proposal these costs would be similar to today's financing in that it would come from employers and increasing excise taxes. Furthermore, control of the rising health care cost would be attempted, thereby saving money.

Personal Responsibility. According to Clinton's stated principles in the Health Care Proposal, personal responsibility refers both to individuals and their families in protecting and promoting health and contributing to cost of care. For the purposes of this article, individual and family responsibility will be addressed.

This is a value based in the first social welfare provisions of the early founders of this country. These values have continued throughout our history. This has been especially true in relationship to families and their care of their elderly member. Findings from the National Long Term Care Survey (Stone and Kemper, 1990) indicated that over three-fourths of the care for elderly adults is provided by spouses and children. Furthermore, this care is usually provided without assistance from formal agencies (Cox, 1993).

Unfortunately, Medicare coverage does not assist families with the care of elder members. Coverage for services and items that would assist elderly to stay in their own homes and communities is restricted (Cox, 1993). For instance, home care, day treatment services, and reimbursements for items such as glasses are seldom reimbursed. Cox (1993) further points out that the current reimbursement system (i.e., DRG's) present risks to frail elderly by encouraging early discharge of patients who may not be able to care for themselves in their own homes. Moreover, this can place extreme burdens on caregivers in families. As stated previously, families often try to care for the elderly in their own homes with little financial, physical or emotional assistance. Typically, caregivers are usually members of the "sandwich" generation, generally women often working outside the home. They have child rearing duties along with the additional responsibilities of caregiving to an elderly parent or relative. These combined responsibilities often lead to roleoverload, stress and depression.

Under the Clinton proposal, families would be assisted in caring for older family members outside of nursing homes. This is a major positive step forward. It is well known that care within the home is preferred when possible. In addition, home care is much less expensive than nursing home care. This provision could provide the necessary financial support to the family which in turn could increase the emotional well-being of the older persons and their families.

A second area of concern is for individual's to take responsibility for their own health. Generally, individuals, regardless of age should take responsibility for their health and engage in positive health behaviors. However, there have been controversies as to whether personal health practices significantly affect the health status of older adults. For instance, in the 1980's, arguments that health status of the elderly represent the cumulative effect of past behaviors, not current behaviors, were put forth by researchers. Some questioned if large scale efforts aimed at promoting healthy life-styles among the aged could be expected to delay the onset of disease, disability, or death. Others stated that positive health practices can postpone disease and subsequent death. In a study that examined current health behaviors of elderly, those that engaged in positive behaviors were more likely to have less depression, fewer or no physical disabilities, higher self-esteem and fewer or no symptoms of aging (Hawkins, Duncan & McDermott, 1988). While controversies exist in this area, it would seem that the goal of promoting positive health practices of elderly adults is an important one. Unfortunately, the provision of health promotion is virtually nonexistent in the Medicare legislation. Furthermore, under the current financial limitations, adding these provisions does not seem likely.

By maintaining the current Medicare system, health promotion and prevention services would remain nonexistent. Therefore, provisions to support and encourage individual older adults in undertaking positive health practices would not occur. It must be pointed out that these provisions are provided in the proposed plan for all other plans. Again, a two-tier system would prevail.

Inter-Generational Justice. The United States has come to a major crossroad in health care policy. We pay more than any other industrialized nation, with the quality of care equal or less than those nations. As the years have continued we have found more Americans receiving less for their dollars. Many Americans cannot afford health care at all. In this deterioration, the one group that has had universal coverage has been those persons over the age of 65. With the legislation as proposed, the major inequity of lack of health care coverage for those under 65 would be addressed. However, if those persons currently over 65 would be required to stay on Medicare, inequity would again occur. As stated earlier, Medicare does provide universal coverage. However, there are major problems with this system. It would appear that many of these problems would be addressed if those 65 and older were allowed to choose other health care plans, therefore, receiving equal coverage with those under the age of 65. This one area alone, defies the value of inter-generational justice.

Wise Allocation of Resources. Most Americans would agree that there should be universal, high quality health care for all of our citizens. However, when the question of "who pays the bill" is discussed, disagreement resounds. As Stoline and Weiner (1993) state "taxpayers want to pay lower taxes; purchasers seek lower premiums; and patients want the best health care, which may not be the least expensive or most efficient." This move to contain health care cost has greatly impacted current funding for Medicare. For instance, Congress and the Bush Administration agreed to cut $43 billion in the Medicare between 1991 and 1995. Sixteen percent of federal spending reductions in the last decade have come from Medicare even though it represents only 7 percent of the total federal budget (Stoline & Weiner, 1993). Ginsburg and Prout (1990) state that "Medicare is suffering from the paradox of being clinically able, but financially unable, to fulfill its mission of caring for those in need" (p. 644).

Though our country spends almost one of every seven dollars on health care, there are more than 37 million Americans not covered by health insurance. In addition, there are another 25 million people in our country without adequate health insurance. To provide the comprehensive coverage for all Americans, the Health Security proposal states that the funding will continue to come from employer and employee contributions. The Administration plan calls for the following:

- ask all employers and the 30 million Americans who work for them but do not have health care coverage to contribute to their health care;
- increase excise taxes on tobacco and require small contributions from large corporations who chose to form their own health alliance;
- limit the growth in federal health care programs (Medicare, Medicaid . . .).

CONCLUSION

Our health care system is broken. The Administration's proposal as now presented will be unable to fix it according to its present funding formula. In its final form the Health Security plan still may have serious inadequacies, but it is a start. It is encouraging that the basic values and principles underlying this proposal will be validated to a greater degree than those in today's health care system. It is hoped that as new options for plans emerge, ethical considerations will continue to be debated and will affect positive changes.

REFERENCES

American Association of Retired Persons. (November 10, 1993). Board of Directors Document.

Cox, C. (1993). *The Frail Elderly: Problems, Needs, and Community Responses.* CT: Auburn House.

Ginsburg, J. & Prout, D. (1990). Access to health care. *Annals of Internal Medicine*, 112(9), 641-61.

Hawkins, W., Duncan, D., & McDermott, R. (1988). A health assessment of older Americans: Some multidimensional measures. *Preventive Medicine*, 17, 344-356.

Monk, A. (1990). *Health Care of the Aged: Needs, Policies, and Services.* New York: The Haworth Press, Inc.

Preliminary Draft of the Presidents Health Reform Proposal. Washington, DC, September 7, 1993.

Stone, R., and Kemper, P. (1990). *Spouses and children of disabled elders: How large a constituency for long care reform. The Milbank Quarterly*, 67, 485-506.

Stoline, A. & Weiner, J. (1993). *The New Medical Marketplace: A Physician's Guide to the Health Care System in the 1990's.* Baltimore: Johns Hopkins Press.

White House Domestic Policy Council. (1993). *Health Security: The President's Report to the American People.*

Should Medical Care Be a *Right* Without Restrictions by Cost, Age, Citizenship, Prognosis, or Self-Infliction

David C. Blake

The title of this paper represents, in rough outline, *the* moral issue underlying all proposals and plans to reform American health care. This question has not, however, surfaced for any sustained consideration in most of the debates and public forums surrounding health care reform. Perhaps, the reason why is that this question represents not a single issue but a whole complex of issues, many of which would surely challenge our abilities to conduct rational public debates. In the interest of nudging this complex of issues a little closer to the surface of public debate, I would like to note two of the specific issues embodied in the above title, and then focus my remarks on just one of the two.

The two issues are as follows: (1) do only American *citizens* have a moral claim on the health care soon to be guaranteed by the U.S. government; and (2) do those who will have legally guaranteed access to health care also have a *right* (moral or otherwise) to whatever treatment they want . . . "no matter what"? I have a few "observations"–no systematic remarks–to offer on the first ques-

David C. Blake, PhD, JD, is Director, Bioethics Institute of Saint John's Hospital and Health Center and Loyola Marymount University, Santa Monica, CA.

[Haworth co-indexing entry note]: "Should Medical Care Be a *Right* Without Restrictions by Cost, Age, Citizenship, Prognosis, or Self-Infliction?" Blake, David C. Co-published simultaneously in *Activities, Adaptation & Aging* (The Haworth Press, Inc.) Vol. 18, No. 3/4, 1994, pp. 107-121; and: *Ethics and Values in Long Term Health Care* (ed: Patricia J. Villani) The Haworth Press, Inc., 1994, pp. 107-121. Multiple copies of this article/chapter may be purchased from The Haworth Document Delivery Center [1-800-3-HAWORTH; 9:00 a.m. - 5:00 p.m. (EST)].

tion, before I turn my attention to the second. What I am most interested in addressing is whether we can limit on moral grounds–meaning "do we have the intellectual or cultural wherewithal to limit on grounds having to do with what is good and right"–a presumed legal entitlement to health care. My agenda is simply to wonder whether it would be dangerous or imprudent for us to acknowledge an entitlement to health care before we are sure that we can effectively limit the entitlement. Otherwise, the agenda of health care reform, put in place to save us–as a society–from bankrupting ourselves in health care costs, might itself be an accelerating catalyst of this very danger.

Of course, it seems as if we have already acknowledged this right–or something like it. This is, in fact, my first observation on the question about whether only *citizens* should be guaranteed access. It seems rather remarkable how quickly we have gone from debating whether it would be proper for an institution like *government*, in creating statutory entitlements, to guarantee access to health care, to debating about what is the most economically viable plan for achieving this goal. It seems that "yesterday" the health care debate was about *ends* and "today" it is about *means*. "Yesterday," the debate was about whether it would be proper for government to set the good of health care as one of its proper ends; whereas "today" the debate is about what means the U.S. government might follow to secure this end. Of course, it could be that because the Clinton Administration, especially under the leadership of Hillary Rodham Clinton, no longer questioned the goal of universal access, the rest of us fell into place and began talking only about the means. It could also be that we Americans have undergone, in this regard, some profound ideological transformation. Perhaps like Paul on the road to Damascus, we have gone from free-market individualists to government-oriented collectivists.

Surely, neither of these "explanations" is correct. I suspect, rather, that we have suddenly become focused on the question of means because we were simply and finally struck by how "unseemly" it is that so many American citizens go without any or adequate health care. I also suspect that there is operating here the distinctive American proclivity that Robert Bellah and colleagues documented so nicely some years ago in *Habits of the Heart* (1986). Being a highly practical or task-oriented people, it is much more natural for Americans to puzzle out the way to get something than to muse about whether the thing we are going to get is really any good. Bellah and his colleagues put it this way: "For most of us, it is easier to think about how to get what we want than to know what exactly we should want" (Bellah et al., 1986, p. 21). Given this proclivity, it could be that once the *intuition* took hold of our minds that it is unseemly for so many American citizens to go without health care, we collectively grabbed at the chance to talk means.

Be this as it may, I do not think this intuition extends to non-citizens or other peoples. I do not think most Americans find it unseemly that undocumented aliens may not get much or any health care, or that peoples in the so-called "third world" live with little or no health care. I suspect most Americans would find this "unfortunate" or "a shame," but not, intuitively speaking, on a moral par with so many American citizens without health care. My point here, which I would like to offer without any further explanation or argument, is that we may have no *reasons* for extending health care access to non-citizens because we actually have no *reasons* for the current drive to cover all citizens. Instead of being based upon some well-defined and generally accepted conception of health care as a human good that government must guarantee, the apparent consensus over the need for national health care may be grounded in only a moral intuition, and an intuition that applies to some humans but not others.

Allow me now to turn to that second question about limits to a presumed right to health care.

If American citizens were to ask ourselves whether an entitlement to health care is in fact a right to whatever treatment we might want, no matter what the costs and no matter what our condition, I am sure that we would say "of course, not!" Most might actually think it silly to even ask the question. There are, however, two little pieces of American health care history–one much more recent than the other–that make this question not only serious but problematic. The first is what has happened to the patient's right to refuse medical treatment since its initial legal and philosophical formulations in the 1960's and 1970's. A right that was originally thought of as pertaining to dying patients trying to deal with an immanent end of their lives is now a right of unlimited application and effect. In

California, for example, a competent adult patient now has a right to refuse any treatment, under any circumstances, for any reason, and regardless of any consequence (*Thor v. Superior Court of Solano County*, 1993 WL 275260, 8 (Cal.), ___Cal.Rptr.___(1993)). Moreover, this unlimited right to refuse treatment is often the fulcrum for many persuasive arguments to legalize voluntary active euthanasia. For example, if a suicide has a legal right to refuse nutrition and hydration for the apparent purpose of committing suicide, why should not a terminally ill cancer patient also have a legal right to *active* means for ending her life? Thus, what was once a right of supposedly limited application and implication–the terminally ill patient's right to *refuse* intrusive, disproportionate treatment–is now a dramatically comprehensive right.

The second piece of history is as recent as yesterday's newspapers. On September 24, 1993, the *New York Times* first reported the case of a conflict between a hospital in the Virginia suburbs of Washington, D.C. and the mother of an eleven month old anencephalic infant (*In The Matter of Baby K*, U.S. District Court, Eastern District of Virginia, No. 93-68-A, July 1, 1993). The mother decided on an aggressive course of treatment for the child because of her firm Christian belief that all life must be protected. This meant repeated visits to the hospital's pediatric intensive care unit to deal with the infant's recurring respiratory crises. Finally, the hospital said "enough" and sought a court determination–a declaratory judgment–that it could refuse to admit the child the next time the child experienced a medical crisis. Among other things, a federal district judge ruled that such a refusal would violate not only the child's right under the Americans with Disabilities Act (ADA) (42 U.S.C. Secs. 120101 et.seq.) but also the mother's right under the Fourteenth Amendment to raise the child the way she thinks is best. While this case is certainly not final and might be of little value as a legal precedent, it does seem to illustrate the possible difficulty of limiting, even in the most hopeless of cases, a right to health care once established.

Of course, some might find fault for the bringing of the issue of patients refusing treatment into the discussion of an entitlement health care. There is, after all, a longstanding distinction within both American jurisprudence and American political philosophy, between a right to be left alone and an entitlement to public assistance. In this jurisprudence and philosophy, the rules and principles behind the "negative" right are not meant to apply to the "positive" right. For example, I cannot infer that you owe me–as a matter of law–assistance when I am in need from the legal rule that you are prohibited from interfering with my lawful conduct. Moreover, I am sure that many would also argue that the Virginia Federal District Court ruling is an aberration, both in regards to how the ADA is supposed to work in the healthcare setting and how the Fourteenth Amendment should be read in terms of parents' rights to raise their children.

I would agree to this response if it were not for the operation, in our jurisprudence on the right to refuse medical treatment, of a profound, culturally-based presumption that could easily work its way into the question of limits to an entitlement to health care. And this presumption is, I suspect, operating in the Virginia anencephalic case.

The reason that we have a right to refuse treatment is that the courts have found in two prominent traditions of American Law analogs for the health care setting. The first is the Common Law Tradition in which courts have, on their own initiative, recognized a legally protected interest that every citizen has in his or her own physical security. This is the Common Law right to physical security; a right that when violated in acts of battery and/or assault gives rise to civil liability (in addition to any criminal liability) on the part of the person violating the right. The second tradition is our history of Constitutional Law, in which protection from governmental interference is extended to various kinds of "private" or "personal" activity, except where there are compelling state interests necessitating and justifying some narrow restriction of the activity. This is the inferred constitutional right of privacy or the 14th Amendment constitutional right of liberty.

In the health care setting, these older and broader rights give birth to a right to refuse treatment. Since medical treatment is an invasion of one's bodily integrity and since the decision to treat or not is properly a matter of one's privacy or a liberty interest, any patient has a legal right to *decide* to *refuse* treatment. This common law and constitutional right to refuse medical treatment cannot, of course, be unlimited *in* principle. Ours is a system of "ordered liberty," meaning the rights of individuals may always be limited or circumscribed, if there is a compelling enough interest that can be furthered in a way that limits the right as little as possible. Thus, the reason why we now have a right to refuse medical treatment that is *practically unlimited* has to do with how the courts have analyzed and ruled on various possible state interests that might limit or circumscribe this particular right.

Typically, courts identify four interests that *might* justify some state restrictions on a patient's right to refuse treatment: (1) the preservation of human life or the dignity of human life; (2) the preservation of the ethical integrity of medicine; (3) the prevention of suicide; and (4) the protection of third-party interests (Blake, 1989). In applying these interests to individual cases where a patient or her surrogate is attempting to refuse treatment, the firmly established legal precedent is that these interests do not limit or circumscribe, in any way, the exercise of this right. The one exception to this clear precedent are a very few cases wherein the interest of dependent minor children ("third parties" to the physician-patient relationship) is considered strong enough to authorize treatment against the patient's (i.e., parent's) wishes.

In order to illustrate how the courts have arrived at this precedent, I would like to offer what I consider to be a representative sampling of the kind of analysis that the courts have exercised over these interests. I will focus on the first two mentioned: human life and medicine's ethical integrity, since the fourth interest is an exception to this precedent, as already mentioned, and the third interest is not considered relevant whenever death following the termination of treatment can be attributed to some underlying medical or physical condition (e.g., cancer, AIDS).

In regards to a state interest in human life limiting a patient's right to refuse treatment, the Massachusetts Supreme Court asserts the following:

> The constitutional right to privacy, as we conceive it, is an expression of the sanctity of individual free choice and self-determination as fundamental constituents of life. The value of life as so perceived is lessened not by a decision to refuse treatment, but by the failure to allow a competent human being the right of choice. (*Superintendent of Belchertown v. Saikewicz*, 373 Mass. 728, 370 N.E.2d 417 (1977), 426)

It seems then that the value of human life is a function of the individual exercising control over that life and thus its value. This court would not, of course, explicitly assert that a live patient who has lost the capacity for choice or self-determination no longer has a life worthy of any state interest. This court does, however, seem to see no possible conflict between a right to refuse treatment and a state interest in preserving the value of human life, since the individual and not the state will get to say if and when his or her life is worth protecting.

This interpretation seems confirmed by the New Jersey Supreme Court's analysis of this matter:

> While. . . [the state interest in preserving the life of the particular patient and in preserving the sanctity of life] . . . are certainly strong, in themselves they will usually not foreclose a competent person from declining life sustaining medical treatment for himself. This is because the life that the state is seeking to protect in such a situation is the life of the same person who has competently decided to forego the medical intervention; it is not some other actual or potential life that cannot adequately protect itself. (*In re Conroy*, 98 N.J. 321, 486 A.2d 1209 (1985), 1223)

Thus, the state apparently has no interest in protecting an individual against her own negative assessment of the value of her life. The state will only protect against someone else's negative assessment of that life.

Again, the Massachusetts Supreme Court in yet another case:

> The duty of the State to preserve life must encompass a recognition of an individual's right to avoid circumstances in which the individual himself would feel that efforts to sustain life demean or degrade his humanity . . . It is antithetical to our scheme of ordered liberty and to our respect for the autonomy of the individual for the state to make decisions regarding the individual's quality of life. It is for the patient to decide such issues. (*Brophy v. New England Sinai Hosp. Inc.*, 398 Mass. 417, 497 N.E.2d 626 (1986), 635)

Thus, for the public to respect the autonomy of some individual the public must not form judgments about the value of her life, even if those judgments would vest more value in her life than she would.

In the rather well-publicized case of Elizabeth Bouvia, the young quadriplegic with a reputed intent to starve herself to death, a California Court of Appeals seems to follow suit in its analysis of this state interest.

> [Elizabeth Bouvia], as the patient, lying helplessly in bed, unable to care for herself, may consider her existence meaningless. She cannot be faulted for so concluding. If her right to choose may not be exercised because there remains to her, in the opinion of a court, a physician or some committee, a certain arbitrary number of years, months, or days, her right will have lost its value and meaning. (*Bouvia v. Superior Court (Glenchur)*, 179 Cal.App.3d 1127, 225 Cal. Rptr. 297 (Ct. App. 1986), 304-05)

Thus, Elizabeth Bouvia's right to refuse treatment, when analyzed with the state interest in preserving the value of human life, turns out to be a right to be the sole assessor of the value of her life.

This same line of reasoning also seems to operate in regards to the state interest in medicine's ethical integrity. In regards to this state interest, the Massachusetts Supreme Court argues as follows:

> Recognition of the right to refuse treatment . . . does not threaten either the integrity of the medical profession, the proper role of hospitals in caring for such patients or the State's interest in protecting the same. It is not necessary to deny a right of self-determination to a patient in order to recognize the *interests* of doctors, hospitals, and medical personnel in attendance on the patient. (*Superintendent of Belchertown v. Saikewicz, supra.* 426-27, emphasis added)

Notice how the interest of the *state* in the integrity of medicine gets transformed into simply an interest of *doctors* themselves. Thus, the possible conflict between an individual's right and a public concern becomes, under this analysis, a possible conflict between the interests of more or less private parties.

A California appellate court performs this same transformation:

... if the right of the patient to self-determination as to his own medical treatment is to have any meaning at all, it must be paramount to the *interests* of the patient's hospital and doctors. The right of a competent adult patient to refuse medical treatment is a constitutionally guaranteed right which must not be abridged. (*Bartling v. Superior Ct. (Glendale Adventist Med. Ctr.)*, 163 Cal. App. 3d 186, 209 Cal. Rptr. 220 (Ct. App. 1984), 225, emphasis added)

Unfortunately, the court does not explain why the patient's right "must be" paramount to this interest except to imply by its description that this state interest is really a *special* interest of a particular profession.

The Massachusetts Supreme Court takes this notion of medicine's integrity being a matter of the physician's own, possibly private, interest and draws an obvious inference. An individual physician's integrity could not be undermined so long as the court does not compel anyone in particular to comply with a patient's right to refuse treatment.

... we conclude also that, so long as we decline to force the hospital to participate in removing or clamping Brophy's G-tube, there is no violation of the integrity of the medical profession. (*Brophy v. New England Sinai Hosp., Inc., supra.* 638)

A right to refuse treatment is then perfectly compatible with medicine's ethical integrity so long as someone in medicine is willing, as a matter of personal conscience, to carry out the patient's wishes. Thus, asking medicine to comply with a patient's request is not an assault on medicine's integrity so long as there is some physician whose own personal integrity will allow her to go along with the patient's request.

Finally, in analyzing the wishes of a quadriplegic prisoner refusing to take any nourishment from prisoner medical personnel, the California Superior Court addresses the state interest in the ethical integrity of medicine by finding that medicine fulfills its moral duties simply by empowering the patient's choices.

... these standards ... [of medical ethics] ... cannot exist in a social and moral vacuum, thereby encouraging a form of medical paternalism under which the physician's determination of what is "best," i.e., medically desirable, controls patient autonomy. Doctors have the responsibility to advise patients fully of those matters relevant and necessary to making a voluntary and intelligent choice. Once that obligation is fulfilled, if the patient rejected the doctor's advice, the onus of that decision would rest on the patient, not the doctor. (*Thor v. Superior Court of Solono County, supra.*, 7)

The court seems hard pressed to see in medicine's integrity any content other than enabling patients to make their own choices about medical treatment decisions.

The culturally-based presumption that I find operating in this analysis is that all goods–or at least those goods thought to be in some sense "moral"–are not capable of *public* evaluation. Moral goods belong to our private lives and not our public lives. They represent private but not public values. Thus, when the courts are asked to discuss apparent moral goods like human life or medicine's ethical integrity, this culturally-based presumption causes the courts to assign to someone's private life the evaluations of these goods. In the case of the good of human life, each patient–in the context of her private life–gets to assign the value to this good. In the case of medicine's ethical integrity, the same presumption operates when the courts let individual physicians decide for themselves as individuals whether to comply with a patient's wish to forgo treatment.

Another way to make this point would be to say that, for example, in regards to the state interest in human life, we have a good for which there is no credible *public or communal value* to be defended in the face of a patient's refusal of treatment. The court will not allow a public or communal valuing of Elizabeth Bouvia's life, over and above whatever value she assigns to it and in defense of which we will limit what Ms. Bouvia might be allowed in refusing care. And the same seems to hold true for medicine's ethical integrity. In the court's oven, this professional integrity boils down to the integrity of the individual physician whose value is–once again–personally but not publicly determinable.

Notice that what was called for in understanding these state interests was some sense of public or communal goodness that is other or more than simply the aggregate of personal goods privately evaluated. And notice that the courts seem to have had no sense of such a possibility. It is this attitude–that goods or moral values could not possibly have a distinguishable public or communal price–that might very well spill over into our thinking about access to health care and its limits.

If we think that one's health care or the effect of medical treatment on one's physical condition is on a par with life itself and one's professional integrity, then we might very well be inclined to think that only individuals personally involved can properly determine the value of the treatment at issue. If the patient is herself demanding some treatment, who are we–that is, the public or community–to say that given her condition, or given the treatment's cost, or given any other consideration, the treatment should not be available to her? If she has a legal entitlement to health care, haven't we already established as a matter of law and public policy, in cases involving the *refusal* of treatment, that she alone gets to determine the value of her health needing care? I strongly suspect that operating in the background of the judge's ruling in the Virginia anencephalic case is the view that only the patient's surrogate standing in the place of the patient (in this case, the mother standing in the place of the child) gets to say whether this life or state of health is worth treating. Why else would the judge think that the ADA is meant to mandate treatment of anencephalic infants?

Of course, even if we accept that all goods–including the good of health care–are personal values subject only to private evaluations, there is still a basis for restricting the treatment available to any one patient. This one basis is a strict form of rationing or fixed resource allocation. In this system, a total, national limit to health care costs would be established by some, more or less arbitrary means, and then this fixed set of resources would be equally distributed to everyone eligible for the coverage. Each individual would have the same, limited amount of resources available to her, and when these resources were depleted, each would be denied further treatment. The key here, of course, is that new or continuing treatment could be denied without any appeal, explicitly or implicitly, to some public or communal assessment of the value of the patient's life or health care. This seems to be the sort of universal health care plan that could function given this cultural presumption or bias that goods, such as life or health or health care, are exclusively personal values.

This is not, however, a system of universal health care that I would advocate or care to work in. My own preference would be for almost *any* alternative to this strictly rationed system. It seems to me, however, that any alternative to this kind of system will require us to do something that we have not been able to do in the case of patients refusing treatment; that is, set a public standard for critically evaluating and possibly overruling the individual's own assessment of matters of life and death. If we are to acknowledge an entitlement to health care that does not bankrupt us, then we need to be able to say that human life and human health have a communal value that is determinable by social processes and available to "trump" an individual patient's wish to have even more treatment. While we have not been able to say to some patients refusing treatment "we cannot simply stop treating you and let you die because this would be too unseemly given our communal assessment of the value of your life or health," we need now to be able to say "we cannot give you the treatment you want because to treat you in this way under these circumstances would be unseemly, given our communal assessment of the value of your life and health." Whether we can do this is, of course, my question and worry.

This is the issue or question that is at stake in the current debate over "futile" or "medically inappropriate" treatment. The debate is precisely about whether this determination represents a value judgment that healthcare professionals should be allowed to make about the treatment of their patients. Some participants in this debate argue that the doctrine of futility, as a limitation on patients' rights, should be employed only in the strict, narrow sense of treatment having no possible chance of producing the desired physiological effect ("physiological futility") (Troug, 1992). The point to this position seems to be that any other sense of futility puts healthcare professionals in a position to enforce their values on a patient regarding the patient's own treatment. Most others in this debate are, however, willing to accept the value-laden character of broader senses of "futility" (Schneiderman et al., 1990) (Callahan, 1991). They argue, instead, that the dangers of restricting a patient's preferences by a physician's idiosyncratic values are avoided if a determination of futility represents a community consensus or, at least, a consensus of the medical profession.

There are, in fact, two levels at which "values" can enter into a determination of futility. The first relates to the proper goals of medical treatment. Here "futility" means "unable to secure a proper goal of medicine." It is, of course, a matter of values to say what are the proper goals of medicine. For example, Larry Schneiderman and colleagues propose a "qualitative" sense of "futility":

> ...we propose that any treatment that merely preserves perma-nent unconsciousness or that fails to end total dependence on intensive medical care should be regarded as nonbeneficial and, therefore, futile. (1990, p. 952)

Notice that the assumption here is that whatever else might be a proper goal of medicine, simply sustaining biologic function and/or simply sustaining a total dependence on medicine itself cannot possibly be proper goals.

The second level at which values enter a determination of futility involves the reasonableness of taking chances. Here "futility" means "while the treatment might conceivably achieve a proper goal of medicine, the chances are so remote as to be unreasonable to take." Assessing the reasonableness of chance is, of course, another matter of values. Schneiderman and colleagues propose as a defini-tion of "quantitative futility" the following:

> when physicians conclude (either through personal experi-ence, experiences shared with colleagues, or consideration of reported empiric data) that in the last 100 cases, a medical treatment has been useless, they should regard that treatment futile. (1990, p. 951)

Those like Schneiderman who are promoting the development within medicine of a value-consensus over the proper (or, at least, improper) goals of medicine and over the reasonableness of taking chances on treatment options have, of course, an uphill battle to fight. The hill is as large as it is–to the disadvantage of these propo-nents of futility–because of the cultural bias that moral values are private, not public matters. If this bias fails to be overturned in the futility debate, in the same way it failed to be overturned in the debate about a patient's right to refuse treatment, then Schneiderman and his fellow travelers will fail. This, I fear, will leave us with rationing on purely arbitrary economic grounds as our only way to contain health care costs under a system of universal access.

Allow me to conclude with this final thought. This worry about setting limits to an entitlement to health care need not operate in all possible worlds. There is a world in which I would see no problem with a plan for universal access to health care that entails a right to have all the health care a person wants. This would be a world in which people have a very strong, clear understanding of their own mortality and who see the avoidance of death as no intrinsically good thing. I am reminded here of remarks by Michael Ignatieff in a *New Republic* review entitled "Modern Dying":

> Stoicism, not surprisingly, is an ideal in retreat in the modern world. Until the advent of Pasteurian medicine in the 19th century, stoicism enjoyed a certain prestige: all too often there was no alternative to its virtues of silence and heroic endurance. But now that so much illness has been conquered, stoic acceptance of biological fate is equated with fatalism and passivity. The "last men" [a reference to a future race envisioned by Nietzsche in *Thus Spake Zarathustra*] of modernity have jettison a culture of endurance for a culture of complaint. But the stoic tradition always addressed itself to the question a culture of complaint cannot answer: When should I struggle, and when must I give in? (1988, p. 32)

Even if a culture of complaint cannot address this question, we must; if, that is, we are to sensibly use the health care that we are about to be guaranteed as Americans. Americans must re-learn when to struggle and when to give in.

REFERENCES

Bellah, R. N., Madsen, R., Sullivan, W., Swidler, A., & Tipton, S. M. (1986). *Habits of the Heart: Individualism and Commitment in American Life.* New York: Harper & Row.

Blake, D.C. (1989). State interests in terminating medical treatment. *Hastings Center Report, 19,* 5-13.

Callahan, D. (1991). Medical futility, medical necessity: The problem-without-a-name. *Hastings Center Report, 21*, 30-35.

Ignatieff, M. (1988). Modern dying. *The New Republic, December 26*, 28-33.

Schneiderman, L. J., Jecker, N. S., & Jonsen, A. R. (1990). Medical futility: Its meaning and ethical implications. *Annals of Internal Medicine, 112*, 949-54.

Printed and bound by CPI Group (UK) Ltd, Croydon, CR0 4YY

28/10/2024

01780394-0001